YOGA MIND, BODY & SPIRIT

ALSO BY DONNA FARHI

The Breathing Book

ILLUSTRATIONS BY SONYA ROONEY

An Owl Book
Henry Holt and Company ~ New York

YOGA MIND, BODY & SPIRIT

~

A Return to Wholeness

~

DONNA FARHI

Holt Paperbacks
Henry Holt and Company, LLC
Publishers since 1866
175 Fifth Avenue
New York, New York 10010
www.henryholt.com

A Holt Paperback® and ⓗ ® are registered trademarks
of Henry Holt and Company, LLC.

Distributed in Canada by H. B. Fenn and Company Ltd.

Library of Congress Cataloging-in-Publication Data
Farhi, Donna.
   Yoga mind, body & spirit : a return to wholeness / Donna
Farhi.
     p.   cm.
   ISBN-13: 978-0-8050-5970-0
   ISBN-10: 0-8050-5970-9
   1. Yoga, Hatha. I. Title: Yoga mind, body and spirit. II.
Title.
RA781.7F37   2000
613.7'046—dc21   99-048392

Henry Holt books are available for special promotions
and premiums. For details contact: Director, Special Markets.

First Edition 2000

Illustrations by Sonya Rooney, Christchurch, New Zealand.
Photographs by Mannering and Associates, Christchurch, New Zealand

Printed in the United States of America

13   15   14   12

Contents

Introduction   *xiii*
Acknowledgments   *xvi*

Part One: Groundwork

I. Living Principles   *3*

What Is Yoga?	4
The Ten Living Principles	7
Yamas (Wise Characteristics):	8
∾ *Ahimsa* (Compassion for All Living Things)	8
∾ *Satya* (Commitment to the Truth)	9
∾ *Asteya* (Not Stealing)	10
∾ *Brahmacharya* (Merging with the One)	11
∾ *Aparigraha* (Not Grasping)	12
Niyamas (Codes for Living Soulfully)	12
∾ *Shaucha* (Purity)	12
∾ *Santosha* (Contentment)	13
∾ *Tapas* (Burning Enthusiasm)	13
∾ *Swadhyaya* (Self-Study)	14
∾ *Ishvarapranidhana* (Celebration of the Spiritual)	15
What Are Yoga *Asanas* and Why Practice Them?	16
Practicing with Joyfulness	18

II. The Seven Moving Principles *21*

Introduction	22
The Process of Inquiry	24
Preparing for Your Practice	25
Creating a Practice Space	25
Getting Started	26
Essential Yoga Equipment	27
The Seven Moving Principles	29

1. BREATHE: Let the Breath Move You	29
The First Movement	29
～ Inquiry: *Letting the Breath Move You*	31
～ Inquiry: *Amplifying the Breath*	33
Guiding the Breath: *Ujjayi*	33
～ Inquiry: *Guiding the Breath*	34
The Principle in Practice	34

2. YIELD: Yield to the Earth: Weight and Levity	35
～ Inquiry: *Yielding to the Earth*	37
The Principle in Practice	37

3. RADIATE: Move from the Inside Out: The Human Starfish	38
Three Steps to Mastery	38
～ Inquiry: *The Starfish*	40
～ Inquiry: *Navel Radiation in* Asanas	41
The Principle in Practice	41

4. CENTER: Maintain the Integrity of the Spine: The Central Axis	42
Spinal Curves	42
Spinal Integrity	43
Spinal Elongation and Riding the Breath	45
～ Inquiry: *Finding Your Neutral Spine*	46
～ Inquiry: *Spinal Elongation and Riding the Breath*	46
The Principle in Practice	47

5. SUPPORT: Foundations of Support: Structural Building Blocks	47
～ Inquiry: *The Cascade Effect of the Foundation*	48
The Principle in Practice	49

6. ALIGN: Lines of Force: Alignment and Sequential Flow   49
   ∼ Inquiry: *Following the Line of the Bones*   51
The Principle in Practice   52

7. ENGAGE: Engage the Whole Body: The Democratic Body Community   52

The Cellular System   57
   ∼ Inquiry: *The Cellular Body*   58
The System in Practice   58

The Musculoskeletal System   59
   ∼ Inquiry: *The Mover and the Moved*   60
The System in Practice   61

The Fluid System   61
   ∼ Inquiry: *The Fluidic Body*   63
The System in Practice   64

The Organ System   64
   ∼ Inquiry: *"Organ-ized" Standing / Organ Support*   66
   ∼ Inquiry: *The Organ Body Scan*   67
   ∼ Inquiry: *Moving with Organ Support*   69
The System in Practice   70

The Neuroendocrine System   70
Coccygeal Body   72
Sex Glands (Women)   72
Sex Glands (Men)   73
Adrenal Glands   73
Pancreas   73
Heart   73
Thymus Gland   73
Thyroid Gland   74
Parathyroid Glands   74
Pituitary Gland   74
Pineal Gland   74
   ∼ Inquiry: *The Glandular Body*   75
   ∼ Inquiry: *Glandular Support in* Asana *Practice*   75

Summary: Engaging the Whole Body   76

RETURN: Return the Mind to Original Silence: 77
Developing Clear Perception
   ∼ Inquiry: *Sitting Meditation: Anchoring the Mind in Silence*   79

The Baseline Beginning, the Check-in Finish   80
The Principle in Practice   80

Part Two: The Yoga Asanas

III. The Standing Postures   83

Introduction: How to Practice the *Asanas*   84
Using the Chart Guides   84
Prenatal Considerations   85
Essential Skills   86
Incorporating the Seven Moving Principles   86

The Standing Postures   87
Key Moving Principles for the Standing Postures   88

Essential Skills: 88
Standing Well: Mountain Pose   88
   The Feet: Foundations of Support for the Legs   88
   ∼ Inquiry: *Centering the Weight on the Feet*   88
   The Pelvis: Foundation of Support for the Spine   89
   ∼ Inquiry: *Centering the Pelvis*   89
   The Preparatory Stances   90
   ∼ Inquiry: *Preparatory Stance I*   90
   ∼ Inquiry: *Preparatory Stance II*   91
   The Sitting Bone to Heel Connection   92
   ∼ Inquiry: *Finding the Sitting Bone to Heel Connection*   93
   A Note About the Knees   94

The Standing Postures   94
Spinal Rolls   94
Horseman's Pose (*Utkatasana*)   96
Half-Dog Pose (*Ardha Svanasana*)   97
Triangle Pose (*Trikonasana*)   98
Side-Angle Pose (*Parsvakonasana*)   100
Warrior Pose II (*Virabhadrasana* II)   103
Warrior Pose I (*Virabhadrasana* I)   104
Safe Transitions   106
Flank Pose (*Parsvottanasana*)   106
Revolved Triangle Pose (*Parivrtta Trikonasana*)   108
Half-Moon Pose (*Ardha Chandrasana*)   110
Expanded-Leg Pose (*Prasaritta Padottanasana*)   112

Forward Stretch (*Uttanasana*)   *113*

Standing Twist   *115*

Downward-Facing Dog (*Adho Mukha Svanasana*)   *116*

Upward-Facing Dog (*Urdhva Mukha Svanasana*)   *119*

Four-Limb Stick Pose (*Chaturanga Dandasana*)   *122*

Sun Salutation (Beginner's Variation) (*Suryanamaskar*)   *125*

Sun Salutation (Classic Variation) (*Suryanamaskar*)   *126*

IV. The Sitting Postures—Forward Bends and Twists   *131*

Introduction   *132*

Key Moving Principles for the Forward Bends   *133*

Essential Skills   *133*

Sitting Well: Stick Pose   *133*

The Pelvis: Finding Your Base of Support   *133*

    ～ Inquiry: *Centering the Weight Through the Pelvis*   *134*

Bending Forward: Moving from Your Hips   *135*

Spinal Reach of the Head and Tail   *135*

    ～ Inquiry: *Bending Forward with Ease*   *136*

Descending the Femurs   *136*

    ～ Inquiry: *Descending the Femurs*   *138*

The Forward Bends   *138*

Reclining Big-Toe Pose (*Supta Padangusthasana*)   *138*

Simple Sitting   *141*

Tailor's Pose (*Sukhasana*)   *141*

Sage Pose (*Siddhasana*)   *141*

Cow-Face Pose (*Gomukasana*)   *142*

Head-to-Knee Pose (*Janu Sirsasana*)   *143*

Revolved Head-to-Knee Pose (*Parivrtta Janu Sirsasana*)   *145*

Wide-Spread-Angle Pose I and II (*Upavistha Konasana* I and II)   *146*

Bound-Angle Pose (*Baddha Konasana*)   *148*

Lotus Posture Preparations: *149*

    ～ Growing Your Lotus: The Swan   *150*

    ～ Through-the-Hole Stretch   *150*

    ～ Cradle Stretch   *151*

Half-Lotus Forward Bend (*Ardha Baddha Padma Paschimottanasana*)   *152*

Lotus Pose (*Padmasana*)   *154*

West Stretch (*Paschimottanasana*)   *155*

Boat Pose (*Navasana*)   *156*

Long and Strong Abdominal Warm-up   *156*

The Twists   158
Key Moving Principles for the Twists   158

Essential Skills   158
The Spiral Staircase   158
   ～ Inquiry: *Turning from the Inside Out*   160
Cautions   160
Standing Twist   161
Crossed-Legs Twist (*Parivrtta Siddhasana*)   161
Revolved Belly Pose (*Jathara Parivartanasana*)   162
Sage Pose I and II (*Bharadvajasana* I and II)   164
Marichi Pose I and III (*Marichyasana* I and III)   166
Lord of the Fishes Pose (*Ardha Matsyendrasana*)   169

V. The Back Bends   *171*

Introduction   172
Key Moving Principles for the Back Bends   173

Essential Skills   173
Elongate Before Bending Backward   173
Using the Whole Spine: Mobilizing the Upper Back   173
   ～ Inquiry: *Elongating the Spine Before Extension*   174
Mobilizing the Rigid Areas of the Back   175
Support Your Back from the Front: The Hyoid   176
   ～ Inquiry: *Engaging the Hyoid*   177
   ～ Inquiry: *Back Bending with Frontal Support*   179

Back-Bending Preparatory Stretches: *Opening the Shoulders*   180
The Shoulder Clock   180
Shoulder Chair Stretch   181

Back-Bending Preparatory Stretches: *Opening the Back*   182
Back Bend over a Bolster   182
Back Bend Through a Chair   183
Back Bend over a Ball   185

Back-Bending Preparatory Stretches: *Opening the Groin and Thighs* 187
Warrior Pose I   187
Hero's Pose and Reclining Hero's Pose (*Virasana* and *Supta Virasana*) 188

The Back-Bending Postures   190
Locust Pose (*Salabhasana*)   190

Child's Pose (*Balasana*)   193

Bridge Pose (*Setu Bandhasana*)   194

Bow Pose (*Dhanurasana*)   195

Camel Pose (*Ustrasana*)   196

Cobra Pose (*Bhujangasana* I)   198

Upward-Facing Bow Pose (*Urdhva Dhanurasana*)   200

Releasing the Back After Back Bends   204

VI. Arm Balances and Upside-Down Poses   *205*

Introduction   206

Inversions and Menstruation   207

Key Moving Principles for the Arm Balances and Upside-Down Poses   208

Essential Skills   208

The Hands: Foundations of Support   208

 ～ Inquiry: *The Arms Mirror the Hands*   209

The Head as Central Support   210

Framing the Head   210

 ～ Inquiry: *The Frame of the Head, Neck, and Shoulders*   211

Using the Wall for Support   212

The Arm Balances and Upside-Down Poses   214

One-Arm Stand (*Vasisthasana*)   214

East Stretch (*Purvottanasana*)   214

Handstand (*Adho Mukha Vrksasana*)   216

Elbow Stand (*Pinchamayurasana*)   218

Headstand (*Sirsasana*)   220

Shoulder Stand (*Salamba Sarvangasana*)   223

Plow Pose (*Halasana*)   226

Knee-to-Ear Pose (*Karnapidasana*)   228

VII. Restorative Postures and Breathing Practices   *231*

Introduction   232

Key Moving Principles for the Restoratives   233

Essential Skills   233

Lying Down and Getting Up with Ease   233

 ～ Inquiry: *Lying Down and Getting Up with Ease*   234

Corpse Pose (*Savasana*)   235

 ～ Inquiry: *Corpse Pose*   236

Quiet Eyes . . . Quiet Mind   237
  ∼ Inquiry: *Practicing with the Eye Bag and Eye Bandage*   238

The Restorative Postures   238
Variation on Corpse Pose (with chair)   239
Variation on Corpse Pose (with bolster)   239
Downward-Facing Corpse Pose   239
Supported Forward Bend   240
Breathing-Easy Position   241
Supported Bound-Angle Pose (*Salamba Supta Baddha Konasana*)   243
The Great Rejuvenator (*Viparita Karani*)   245

Breathing Practices   247
Straw Breathing   247
The Purifying Breath (*Nadi Shodhanam*)   248
The Pacifying Breath (*Viloma* II)   249

Part Three: Practice

VIII. Putting It All Together   *253*

Introduction   254
The Alphabet of Yoga *Asanas*: Structural Sequencing   256
General Practice   260
Thematic Practice   260
Transitional Movements and Counterpostures   260
A Core Structure for Any Practice   262

Beginning Sequences   263
  Practice Session A: Rise and Shine   263
  Practice Session B: Opening Up   264
  Practice Session C: Turning Inward   265
  Practice Session D: Returning   265

Intermediate/Advanced Sequences   266
  Practice Session A: Rise and Shine   266
  Practice Session B: Opening Up   267
  Practice Session C: Turning Inward   267
  Practice Session D: Inner Power   268
  Practice Session E: Returning   269

Notes   270

Introduction

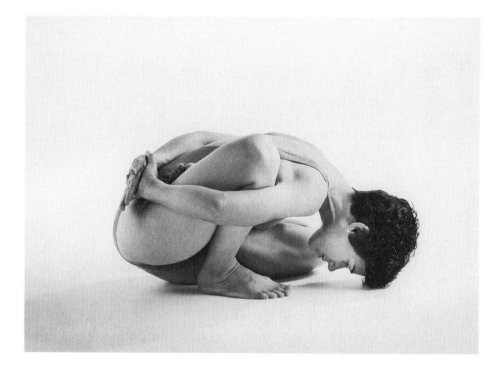

The inner – what is it?
if not intensified sky,
hurled through with birds
and deep with
the winds of homecoming.

—RAINER MARIA RILKE

One of my closest mentors, the late Ray Worring, used to take me on long drives through the wilderness areas of Montana. After one such drive Ray suggested I spend some time looking out over the mountain range. Even though the view was extraordinary, I began to balk at the discomfort of sitting in the freezing wind, numbed to the bone with cold. For what purpose had we come so far simply to sit and look at a mountain? It took many years before I understood the message he wished to impart that early-spring day: You are this vastness. This vista you see, this grandeur, this enduring strength—if you go deeply enough inside yourself, you will find not something small but something immensely spacious. This is the essence of the human spirit. This message, imparted so simply and yet ineffably etched into my experience of myself and the world, had an enormous influence in shaping what I came to see as the purpose of yoga—to reconnect to the original vastness and silence of the mind. And it was integral to Ray's teachings that this understanding of oneself be not only an intellectual idea but a felt cellular experience in the body.

In the early sixties, when yoga became popular through the work of Richard Hittleman and other such luminaries, the teachers of that time had to find a way to make an Eastern science and art palatable to the Western mind. This was no easy task. Most presented yoga's tangible forms—the postures and the more pragmatic breathing exercises. These forms the Western mind could easily grasp. Others presented the esoteric aspects of yoga in teachings that reached few and were understood by even fewer. Form is what the Western mind could understand, and so it was the forms of yoga that were emphasized. In an effort to popularize yoga the more essential spiritual message of the practice has been pared away and oftentimes completely eliminated.

Increasingly doing "good" yoga has come to mean having a beautiful body, remaining forever youthful, and being able to show one's adeptness through the seemingly solid evidence of advanced postures. But as we stretch our muscles deeply or strengthen our abdominals, are we coming closer to feeling a deep peacefulness within ourselves and an inner equanimity that can meet the challenges of life in a compassionate and skillful way? Like the botanist who finally breeds the perfect rose only to discover that in the process he has lost the fragrance of the bloom, when we strip yoga to its mechanics, we also lose something essential. The task of today's teachers and students is to reclaim the essential spirit and intention behind these practices in a way that challenges rather than placates the underpinnings of this Western mind. For it is this change of mind that is so desperately needed to bring about healing in the world today.

I have been as guilty as any of both practicing and teaching yoga in a way that made the postures and practices more important than the spirit of the person practicing them. My early obsession with perfecting the forms of yoga brought with it a greater and greater sense of unease and inner dissatisfaction. The realization that I had bought into the dictum of a culture obsessed with achievement and the unhappiness wrought by such striving led me to a long period of deep experimentation in my own practice. Through the generosity and willingness of my students to join me in this inquiry, I have slowly uncovered a more natural way of discovering the essence of the practice *through* form. The forms then become vehicles for experiencing one's essential nature rather than goals in and of themselves. Then whether you attain any particular posture becomes irrelevant. The shift from dominating, controlling, or ignoring nature to listening and working with nature's wisdom marks the beginning of this change of mind. When we shift from being the mover to letting *life move through us,* we make the first step toward surrendering our heart to spiritual practice. This step marks the beginning of yoga as a life path rather than a form of sophisticated calisthenics. I am convinced that there is nothing new about this approach and that it can best be described as a neoclassical revival of the original way of working first explored by yogis centuries ago. I am equally convinced that anyone who becomes quiet enough to observe the way of nature will arrive at conclusions similar to my own. The ancient teachings of Yoga, and others such as Taoism, Buddhism, and Ayurveda all spring from the same universal source of wisdom.

My teacher, Ray, encouraged me to work with the body in the service of regenerating the connection to the spirit. So this book is my gift to those who would wish to reunite with their spiritual life through the body. Observing, perceiving, feeling, and acting from the wisdom of the natural world is nonetheless a long apprenticeship. Even the very idea of apprenticeship is a foreign one in the face of a society compelled to follow anything that offers immediate gratification. But the slowness of this path *is* part of the healing. It is part of finding one's place in the rhythm of life again. This reunification with nature lies at the heart of the true healing power of yoga practice. Through that practice we can become peaceful, we can experience ease with ourselves and others, and ultimately we can create a society that values such things. Then as we advance in our yoga practice, we will realize that however far we go, we are always in the process of returning to this natural self.

Donna Farhi
May 2000

Acknowledgments

Many people nurture the creation of a book, the least of whom are the poor fellows who must live with the writer through the often difficult and cantankerous period of gestation. My partner, Mark Bouckoms, has been one such fellow, buffeting the thick and the thin of it with me and offering enormous support in the way that only good friends can.

I am tremendously grateful to my past and present mentors and teachers who have, through their own practice and commitment, inspired my love for yoga. Among these are Jim Spira, Judith Lasater, Angela Farmer, Dona Holleman, and many others who were faculty at the time of my training at the Iyengar Yoga Institute in San Francisco. Although I have had few opportunities to study personally with Bonnie Bainbridge Cohen, her writings and teachings as taught through Body-Mind Centering® practitioners and colleagues such as Lynne Uretsky have been central to helping me find a physical language for helping others experience the totality of the body.

My nascent years as a writer for *Yoga Journal* were particularly fostered by one caring editor—Linda Cogozzo. Without her encouragement I daresay I would never have ventured to commit myself to the printed word. The journal itself has throughout my career spurred me to crystallize my thoughts and thus has been a central means of sharing my ongoing research with the worldwide yoga community.

I am personally indebted to my mentor and spiritual teacher, Ray Worring, who died before this manuscript was finished. His message of loving, gifting, and sharing helped me to see that living one's dharma is the ultimate service to others.

My special thanks to Murray Irwin and Pat Dolin of Mannering and Associates in Christchurch for surviving the rigors of a three-day photo shoot that left us all sore and bleary-eyed, and to Mark Bouckoms, Evan Porter, and Tui Short for their time in modeling many of the pictures. The exquisite and inspiring illustrations in this book were created in collaboration with artist Sonya Rooney, who was a delight to work with from start to finish. Books also need their advocates, and one would be hard-pressed to find a better one than my literary agent, Laurie Fox, whose boundless enthusiasm was thankfully matched by the effusive Amelia Lee Sheldon, my editor at Henry Holt. Her thoughtful consideration of the structure and content of this book were priceless. Unsung heroine behind the scenes Lucy Albanese, art director at Holt, has ensured that this book will be not only useful but also beautiful.

Last, my thanks to all the wonderful students who have blessed my life and taught me so much more than any of them could know. Also to the many people at centers and yoga studios throughout the world responsible for sponsoring my teaching visits. And to nature, that great teacher of the way of things.

Part One
~
Groundwork

I
Living Principles

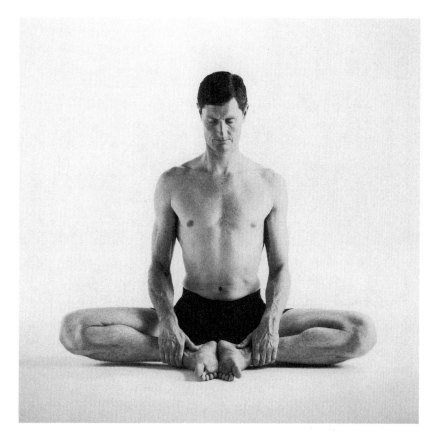

*Any change into a new state of being
is the result of the fullness of Nature
unfolding inherent potential.*

—THE YOGA SUTRAS OF PATANJALI[1]

WHAT IS YOGA?

*A*ll people wish to be happy. This seemingly simple desire appears to elude the best-intentioned efforts of even the most intelligent among us. Yet almost everyone has had glimpses of deep peacefulness when they have felt connected both to themselves, to others, and to nature. Curiously, the state of feeling good and whole does not seem to be something we can order up on demand but rather appears to happen spontaneously. In such moments we experience a sense of translucence such that that which we see, feel, sense, hear, or touch no longer feels separate from us but is experienced as a part of our own totality. When our hand resting over the heart of the beloved merges and becomes one with his or her body, when we become the same midnight sky that fills us with awe, we remember, however briefly, our place in the scheme of things. These brief flickers of remembrance imbue our vision with freshness and innocence so that we can see things as they truly are. Because these moments of lucidity are so blissful, we wish that they may become the base state of our lives rather than the brief and oftentimes tenuous experience to which such happiness is usually assigned. These moments of clarity have nothing to do with the caricatures of happiness presented to us through the media or popular culture. These moments have always been there. The beloved's heartbeat and the sky have always been there. These moments are simply awaiting our arrival.

Yoga is a technology for arriving in this present moment. It is a means of waking up from our spiritual amnesia, so that we can remember all that we *already* know. It is a way of remembering our true nature, which is essentially joyful and peaceful. Developed as a pragmatic science by ancient seers centuries ago, yoga is a practice that any person, regardless of age, sex, race, or religious belief, can use to realize her full potential. It is a means of staying in intimate communication with the formative core matrix of yourself and those forces that serve to bind all living beings together. As you establish and sustain this intimate connection, this state of equanimity becomes the core of your experience rather than the rare exception.

Through observing nature and through intense self-observation and inquiry, the ancient yogis were able to codify the conditions that must be present for realizing our intrinsic wholeness. Although such realization can occur spontaneously, more often than not it is the result of a sustained commitment to practice over a lifetime. This is not to imply that yoga is a goal which we strive toward, or that there is some kind of chronological progression toward "self-improvement." Rather, it is the recognition that each individual can achieve understanding only through his own exploration and discovery, and that all of life is a continual process of refinement which allows us to see more clearly. When we clean the windshield of our car, we suddenly see the road ahead as bright and defined. The road, the image before us, is exactly as it was before we cleaned the window. The trees are the same green, the sky the same vivid blue, and the markers just as defined, only now we see what is there. We start to be able to see the potholes in the road ahead and to avoid them. We start to remember such dangerous roads and steer our way clear to safer routes in the future. In the same way, yoga is not about self-improvement or making ourselves better. It is a process of deconstructing all the barriers we may have erected that prevent us from having an authentic connection with ourselves and with the world. This tenet is an extremely important one because the effort to change and improve ourselves is fraught with the risk of subtle self-aggression that only produces more unhappiness. We cannot strive toward something that we already are.

Nonetheless, there *is* work to be done. And this work is not about following a formula, or strictly adhering to rules, because yoga is not a paint-by-numbers affair. Nor does yoga require blind faith in an outside authority or dogma. Nor is it a religion, although the practice of its central precepts inevitably draws each individual to the direct experience of those truths on which religion rests. Rather, yoga is a way of living and being that makes real happiness possible. Yoga is also a science that incorporates a broad range of practices and techniques that can be tailored and adapted to best suit your personal constitution and personality. We are not asked to believe anything until we have experimented, tested, and found our direct experience to be sound. The great paradox of this "work" is that there is no reward to strive toward, because the practice *is* the reward. In the very moment you focus your attention by coming back into your body, your breath, and your immediate sensate reality, you will experience a deep sense of vibrant stillness. This feeling is so pleasurable, so joyful and revitalizing that you will be drawn to practice, and, more important, you will begin to be naturally drawn toward lifestyle choices that nourish your well-being. This work is not about forcing yourself to give up anything, because that which is no longer nourishing to you will gradually drop away effortlessly. There is no waiting and no delayed gratification because yoga is both the means and the result, and the seed of all that is possible is present at the very beginning. This experience of stillness is possible in the first ten minutes of your first yoga class. It is possible in this very breath. Sadly, if we approach and practice yoga with the same cultural dictum of striving and effort, force and self-coercion that we may have applied to other aspects of our lives, we may practice diligently for decades while never allowing our self to appreciate the simple truth of its own wholeness.

Although there are many branches to the tree of yoga, from devotional methods to more intellectual approaches, from schools that emphasize service toward others to those that focus on physical purification, Patanjali, the author of the Yoga Sutras, clearly defines an eight-limbed path (*ashtanga*) that forms the structural framework for whatever emphasis upon which an individual wishes to concentrate. The Yoga Sutras, or "threads," consist of four books produced sometime in the third century before Christ. Such was the clarity of Patanjali's vision of wholeness that he consolidated the entirety of yoga philosophy in a series of 196 lucid aphorisms. Each thread of the Yoga Sutras is revealed as a part of a woven fabric, with each aphorism merely a mark or color within the whole pattern. The threads, however, begin to make sense only through a direct experience of their meaning. This is not a linear process but rather an organic one in which colors and markings gradually become more clear until a pattern forms. And this pattern that Patanjali weaves for us is a description of the process of unbinding our limited ideas about ourselves and becoming free.

The eight limbs of yoga are traditionally presented as a hierarchical progression, but this linear progression toward an idealized goal tends only to reinforce the dualistic idea that yoga is something to "get." It may be more helpful to imagine the eight limbs as the arms and legs of a body—connected to one another through the central body of yoga. Just as a child's limbs grow in proportion to one another, whatever limb of practice we focus upon inevitably causes the other limbs to grow as well. People who begin yoga through the limb of meditation are often later drawn to practice more physical postures. Those who are drawn to vigorous physical practice later find themselves being drawn into the quieter, more meditative practices. Just as each limb is essential for the optimal functioning of your body, every limb of yoga practice is important. Growth in practice happens naturally when a person is sincere in her wish to grow.

The eight limbs emanating from a central core consist of the following:

Yamas and *Niyamas:* Ten ethical precepts that allow us to be at peace with ourselves, our family, and our community.

Asanas: Dynamic internal dances in the form of postures. These help to keep the body strong, flexible, and relaxed. Their practice strengthens the nervous system and refines our process of inner perception.

Pranayama: Roughly defined as breathing practices, and more specifically defined as practices that help us to develop constancy in the movement of *prana,* or life force.

Pratyahara: The drawing of one's attention toward silence rather than toward things.

Dharana: Focusing attention and cultivating inner perceptual awareness.

Dhyana: Sustaining awareness under all conditions.

Samadhi: The return of the mind into original silence.

The greater part of this book on yoga will focus on the most down-to-earth practices—the *asanas* and the practices of breathing and meditation. These form an embodied approach to spiritual practice, where we use the body and all our sensual capacities in the service of regeneration and transformation. This is contrasted to many approaches in which the body is seen as an obstacle that must be transcended. Let us first look at the core principles for living, the *yamas* and *niyamas* that form the central vein from which all other yoga practices spring.

THE TEN LIVING PRINCIPLES

The first limb, or the *yamas,* consists of characteristics observed and codified by wise people since the beginning of time as being central to any life lived in freedom. They are mostly concerned with how we use our energy in relationship to others and, in a subtler sense, our relationship to ourselves. The sages recognized that stealing from your neighbor was likely to promote discord, lying to your wife would cause suffering, and violence begets more violence; the results are hardly conducive to living a peaceful life. The second limb, the *niyamas,* constitutes a code for living in a way that fosters the soulfulness of the individual and has to do with the choices we make. The *yamas* and *niyamas* are emphatic descriptions of what we *are* when we are connected to our source. Rather than a list of dos and don'ts, they tell us that our fundamental nature is compassionate, generous, honest, and peaceful.[2]

In the West we are taught from an early age that what we do and what we own are the sole components for measuring whether we are "successful." We measure our success and that of others through this limited vantage point, judging and dismissing anything that falls outside these narrow parameters. What yoga teaches us is that *who* we are and *how* we are constitute the ultimate proof of a life lived in freedom. If you do not truly believe this, it is likely that you will measure success in your yoga practice through the achievement of external forms. This tendency has produced a whole subculture of yoga in the West that is nothing more than sophisticated calisthenics, with those who can bend the farthest or do the most extraordinary yoga postures being deemed masters. Because it's easy to measure physical prowess, we may compare ourselves to others who are more flexible, or more "advanced" in their yoga postures, getting trapped in the belief that the forms of the practice *are* the goal. These outward feats do not necessarily constitute any evidence of a balanced practice or a balanced life. What these first central precepts the *yamas* and *niyamas* ask us to remember is that the techniques and forms are not goals in themselves but vehicles for getting to the essence of who we are.

One of our greatest challenges as Westerners practicing yoga is to learn to perceive progress through "invisible" signs, signs that are quite often unacknowledged by the culture at large. Are we moving toward greater kindness, patience, or tolerance toward others? Are we able to remain calm and centered even when others around us become agitated and angry? How we speak, how we treat others, and how we live are more subjective qualities and attributes we need to learn to recognize in ourselves as a testament to our own progress and as gauges of authenticity in our potential teachers. When we remain committed to our most deeply held values we can begin to discern the difference between the *appearance* of achievement and the *true experience* of transformation, and thereby free ourselves to pursue those things of real value.

As you read through the precepts that follow, take the time to dwell upon their relevance to your life and to consider your own personal experiences both past and present in reference to them. You can take almost any situation that arises in your life and consider it from the vantage point of one or more of these precepts. It can also be valuable consciously to choose a precept that you'd like to explore in depth for a month or even a year at a time, investigating how the precept works in all aspects of your life. And last, the way in which you approach the practices that follow in this book, and your underlying intentions, will ultimately determine whether your practice bears fruit. As you progress in your yoga practice, take the time to pause frequently and ask "Who am I becoming through this practice? Am I becoming the kind of person I would like to have as a friend?"

Yamas—Wise Characteristics

Ahimsa—*Compassion for All Living Things*
Ahimsa is usually translated as nonviolence, but this precept goes far and beyond the limited penal sense of not killing others. First and foremost we have to learn how to be nonviolent toward ourselves. If we were able to play back the often unkind, unhelpful, and destructive comments and judgments silently made toward our self in any given day, this may give us some idea of the enormity of the challenge of self-acceptance. If we were to speak these thoughts out loud to another person, we would realize how truly devastating violence to the self can be. In truth,

few of us would dare to be as unkind to others as we are to ourselves. This can be as subtle as the criticism of our body when we look in the mirror in the morning, or when we denigrate our best efforts. Any thought, word, or action that prevents us (or someone else) from growing and living freely is one that is harmful.

Extending this compassion to all living creatures is dependent on our recognition of the underlying unity of all sentient beings. When we begin to recognize that the streams and rivers of the earth are no different from the blood coursing through our arteries, it becomes difficult to remain indifferent to the plight of the world. We naturally find ourselves wanting to protect all living things. It becomes difficult to toss a can into a stream or carve our names in the bark of a tree, for each act would be an act of violence toward ourselves as well.

Cultivating an attitude and mode of behavior of harmlessness does not mean that we no longer feel strong emotions such as anger, jealously, or hatred. Learning to see everything through the eyes of compassion demands that we look at even these aspects of our self with acceptance. Paradoxically, when we welcome our feelings of anger, jealousy, or rage rather than see them as signs of our spiritual failure, we can begin to understand the root causes of these feelings and move beyond them. By getting close enough to our own violent tendencies we can begin to understand the root causes of them and learn to contain these energies for our own well-being and for the protection of others. Underneath these feelings we discover a much stronger desire that we all share—to be loved. It is impossible to come to this deeper understanding if we bypass the tough work of facing our inner demons.

In considering *ahimsa* it's helpful to ask, Are my thoughts, actions, and deeds fostering the growth and well-being of all beings?

Satya—*Commitment to the Truth*

This precept is based on the understanding that honest communication and action form the bedrock of any healthy relationship, community, or government, and that deliberate deception, exaggerations, and mistruths harm others. One of the best ways we can develop this capacity is to practice right speech. This means that when we say something, we are sure of its truth. If we were to follow this precept with commitment, many of us would have a great deal less to say each day! A large part of our everyday comments and conversations are not based upon what we know to be true but are based on our imagination, suppositions, erroneous conclusions, and sometimes out-and-out exaggerations. Gossip is probably the worst form of this miscommunication.

Commitment to the truth isn't always easy, but with practice, it's a great deal less complicated and ultimately less painful than avoidance and self-deception. Proper communication allows us to deal with immediate concerns, taking care of little matters before they become big ones.

Probably the hardest form of this practice is being true to our own heart and inner destiny. Confusion and mistrust of our inner values can make it difficult to know the nature of our heart's desire, but even when we become clear enough to recognize what truth means for us, we may lack the courage and conviction to live our truth. Following what we know to be essential for our growth may mean leaving unhealthy relationships or jobs and taking risks that jeopardize our own comfortable position. It may mean making choices that are not supported by consensual reality or ratified by the outer culture. The truth is rarely convenient. One way we can know we are living the truth is that while our choices may not be easy, at the end of the day we feel at peace with ourselves.

Asteya—*Not Stealing*

Asteya arises out of the understanding that all misappropriation is an expression of a feeling of lack. And this feeling of lack usually comes from a belief that our happiness is contingent on external circumstances and material possessions. Within Western industrialized countries satisfaction can be contingent upon so many improbable conditions and terms that it is not uncommon to spend all of one's time hoping for some better life, and imagining that others (who possess what we do not) have that better life. In constantly looking outside of ourselves for satisfaction, we are less able to appreciate the abundance that already exists. That is what really matters—our health and the riches of our inner life and the joy and love we are able to give and receive from others. It becomes difficult to appreciate that we have hot running water when all we can think about is whether our towels are color-coordinated. How can we appreciate our good fortune in having enough food to eat when we wish we could afford to eat out more often?

The practice of *asteya* asks us to be careful not to take anything that has not been freely given. This can be as subtle as inquiring whether someone is free to speak with us on the phone before we launch into a tirade about our problems. Or reserving our questions after a class for another time, rather than hoarding a teacher's attention long after the official class time has ended. In taking someone's time that may not have been freely given, we are, in effect, stealing. The paradox of practicing *asteya* is that when we relate to others from the vantage point of abundance rather than neediness, we find that others are more generous with us and that life's real treasures begin to flow our way.

This may seem unlikely, so let me share an example. Paul was a medical student and past acquaintance who seemed always to be helping others and sharing his seemingly limited resources. One evening when it became too late for a commute home, I offered Paul my guest room for the night. On awakening in the morning I discovered he had cleaned my refrigerator ("It looked like you'd been busy"). Paul had few financial resources but always seemed to be having wonderful dinner feasts to share with his friends. Later, I found out that he worked late at a local health-food restaurant, and, thankful for the extra hours Paul spent helping out, the owner gave him many of the leftover vegetables, breads, and prepared dishes to take home. When a number of friends joined Paul at a holiday home for a week, Paul initiated a special "clean-up and dust" party that lasted all day ("Just think how great it will be for the owner when he comes back after his trip overseas . . ."). Paul rarely asked for anything but was always surprising his friends with his new acquisitions. People gave things to Paul all the time—even large items like cars and washing machines—not because they felt sorry for him but because his own sense of intrinsic abundance and his own generosity tended to make you feel that, like him, you had a lot to give.

Not stealing demands that we cultivate a certain level of self-sufficiency so that we do not demand more of others, our family, or our community than we need. It means that we don't take any more than we need, because that would be taking from others. A helpful way of practicing *asteya* when you find yourself dwelling on the "not enoughs" of your life is to ask: "How is this attitude preventing me from enjoying the things I already have?" Another way of fostering this sense of abundance is to take a moment before going to sleep to dwell on at least one gift in your life. This can be as simple as the gift of having a loving partner or loyal pet, the grace of having good health, or the pleasure of having a garden.

Brahmacharya—*Merging with the One*

Of all the precepts, the call to *brahmacharya* is the least understood and the most feared by Westerners. Commonly translated as celibacy, this precept wreaks havoc in the minds and lives of those who interpret *brahmacharya* as a necessary act of sexual suppression or sublimation. All spiritual traditions and religions have wrestled with the dilemma of how to use sexual energy wisely. Practicing *brahmacharya* means that we use our sexual energy to regenerate our connection to our spiritual self. It also means that we don't use this energy in any way that might harm another. It doesn't take a genius to recognize that manipulating and using others sexually creates a host of bad feelings, with the top contenders being pain, jealousy, attachment, resentment, and blinding hatred. This is one realm of human experience that is guaranteed to bring out the best and worst in people, so the ancient yogis went to great lengths to observe and experiment with this particular form of energy. It may be easier to understand *brahmacharya* if we remove the sexual designation and look at it purely as energy. *Brahmacharya* means merging one's energy with God. While the communion we may experience through making love with another gives us one of the clearest experiences of this meshing of energies, this experience is meant to be extended beyond discrete events into a way of life—a kind of omnidimensional celebration of Eros in all its forms. Whether we achieve this through feeling our breath as it caresses our lungs, through orgasm, or through celibacy is not important.

Given the pragmatism of the ancient yogis, it is hard to believe that Patanjali would have put forth a precept that would be so undeniably unsuccessful as self-willed denial. The fall from grace of countless gurus who, while admonishing their devotees to practice celibacy, have wantonly misused their own sexual power gives cause to consider more deeply the appropriateness of such an interpretation. When any energy is sublimated or suppressed, it has the tendency to backfire, expressing itself in life-negating ways. This is not to say that celibacy in and of itself is an unsound practice. When embraced joyfully the containment of sexual energy can be enormously self-nourishing and vitalizing and, at the very least, can provide an opportunity to learn how to use this energy wisely. When celibacy is practiced in this way, there is no sense of stopping oneself from doing or having what one really wants. Ultimately it is not a matter of *whether* we use our sexual energy but *how* we use it.

In looking at your own relationship to sexual energy, consider whether the ways you express that energy bring you closer to or farther away from your spiritual self.

Aparigraha—*Not Grasping*

Holding on to things and being free are two mutually exclusive states. The ordinary mind is constantly manipulating reality to get ground underneath it, building more and more concretized images of how things are and how others are, as a way of generating confidence and security. We build self-images and construct concepts and paradigms that feed our sense of certainty, and we then defend this edifice by bending every situation to reinforce our certainty. This would be fine if life were indeed a homogeneous event in which nothing ever changed; but life does change, and it demands that we adapt and change with it. The resistance to change, and tenaciously holding on to things, causes great suffering and prevents us from growing and living life in a more vital and pleasurable way. What yoga philosophy and all the great Buddhist teachings tells us is that solidity is a creation of the ordinary mind and that there never was anything permanent to begin with that we could hold on to. Life would be much easier and substantially less painful if we lived with the knowledge of impermanence as the only constant. As we all have discovered at some time in our lives, whenever we have tried to hold on too tightly to anything, whether it be possessiveness of our partner or our youthful identity, this has only led to the destruction of those very things we most value. Our best security lies in taking down our fences and barricades and allowing ourselves to grow, and through that growth becoming stronger and yet more resilient.

The practice of *aparigraha* also requires that we look at the way we use things to reinforce our sense of identity. The executive ego loves to believe in its own power but unfortunately requires a retinue of foot soldiers in the way of external objects such as the right clothes, car, house, job, or image to maintain this illusion. Because this executive ego is but an illusion created by our sense of separateness, it requires ever greater and more elaborate strategies to keep it clothed. Although the practice of not grasping may first begin as consciously withdrawing our hand from reaching for external things, eventually the need to reach outward at all diminishes until there is a recognition that that which is essential to us is already at hand.

Niyamas—Codes for Living Soulfully

Shaucha—*Purity*

Shaucha, or living purely, involves maintaining a cleanliness in body, mind, and environment so that we can experience ourselves at a higher resolution. The word pure comes from the Latin *purus,* which means clean and unadulterated. When we take in healthy food, untainted by pesticides and unnatural additives, the body starts to function more smoothly. When we read books that elevate our consciousness, see movies that inspire, and associate with gentle people, we are feeding the mind in a way that nourishes our own peacefulness. Creating a home environment that is elegant, simple, and uncluttered generates an atmosphere where we are not constantly distracted by the paraphernalia of yesterday's projects and last year's knick-knacks. *Shaucha* is a testament to the positive power of association.

Practicing *shaucha,* meaning "that and nothing else," involves making choices about what you want and don't want in your life. Far from self-deprivation or dry piety, the practice of *shaucha* allows you to experience life more vividly. A clean palate enjoys the sweetness of an apple and the taste of pure water; a clear mind can appreciate the beauty of poetry and the wisdom imparted in a story; a polished table reveals the deep grain of the wood. This practice both generates beauty and allows us to appreciate it in all its many forms.

Santosha—*Contentment*

Santosha, or the practice of *content-ment,* is the ability to feel satisfied within the container of one's immediate experience. Contentment shouldn't be confused with happiness, for we can be in difficult, even painful circumstances and still find some semblance of contentment if we are able to see things as they are without the conflictual pull of our expectations. Contentment also should not be confused with complacency, in which we allow ourselves to stagnate in our growth. Rather it is a sign that we are at peace with whatever stage of growth we are in and the circumstances we find ourselves in. This doesn't mean that we accept or tolerate unhealthy relationships or working conditions. But it may mean that we practice patience and attempt to live as best we can within our situation until we are able to better our conditions.

Contentment not only implies acceptance of the present but tends to generate the capacity for hopefulness. This may seem contradictory but is not. When you are equanimous within any situation, this strengthens your faith that there is the possibility of living even more fully. This possibility is not held out as something to look forward to, nor does it have the negative effect of making you feel dissatisfied until those hopes are gratified. Rather, the ability to sustain one's spirits, even in dire situations, is proof that a central sense of balance is rarely contingent on circumstances. And, sustaining hopefulness, even when there are few signs that things will improve, is one very good way of fostering contentment.

Tapas—*Burning Enthusiasm*

Literally translated as "fire" or "heat," *tapas* is the disciplined use of our energy. Because the word *discipline* has the negative connotation of self-coercion, I take the liberty here of translating this central precept as "burning enthusiasm." When we can generate an attitude of burning ardor, the strength of our convictions generates a momentum that carries us forward. We all know how even a seemingly boring or unpleasant task like cleaning the house can be transformed when we work with vigor and impulsion. Suddenly cleaning the toilet becomes fun, hauling heavy loads invigorating, and dusting the furniture absorbing. *Tapas* is a way of directing our energy. Like a focused beam of light cutting through the dark, *tapas* keeps us on track so that we don't waste our time and energy on superfluous or trivial matters. When this energy is strong, so also are the processes of transmutation and metamorphism.

We are not all equally possessed of the disciplined energy of *tapas.* Some people need to work more earnestly to kindle the flames of *tapas,* and it is at these times that it is helpful to have a kind of parental consciousness coupled with a good sense of humor. Our actions are then guided by a part of the self that knows what's good for it, which is aided by the ability to laugh in the face of one's neuroses, lethargy, or addictions. Even the laser minds among us have days when it takes a sheer act of will to get out of bed, turn to our studies, or withdraw the hand that reaches for a second slice of cake. If you have little enthusiasm yourself, it can be enormously helpful to seek the company of those who have this quality in abundance. Attending a class with an inspiring teacher or practicing yoga with a friend who has already established a strong practice can help to stimulate *tapas* within yourself. Once activated, however, the embers of *tapas* tend to generate more and more heat and momentum, which makes each subsequent effort less difficult. The analogy of a fire is fitting for this precept. Once a fire has completely died out it can take a great deal of effort to start it up again. When you do get a fire to light, the tentative embers must be fed at regular intervals or the fire dies out again. But once the fire is roaring, it is easy to sustain.

For what greater purpose do we need *tapas*, or discipline? Pema Chödrön, the Abbot of Gampo Abbey in Cape Breton, Nova Scotia, and the author of many books on Tibetan Buddhism, tells us that "what we discipline is not our 'badness' or our 'wrongness.' What we discipline is *any form of potential escape from reality*"[3] (italics added). When we're not living in this disciplined awareness, our willing tactics of avoidance create an endless cycle of more suffering for ourselves. These avoidance tactics may temporarily placate our senses, but they create a deep form of unhappiness. On some level we know we're not being true to ourselves or our potential. Discipline is having enough respect for yourself to make choices that truly nourish your well-being and provide opportunities for expansive growth. Far from being a kind of medicinal punishment, *tapas* allows us to direct our energy toward a fulfilled life of meaning and one that is exciting and pleasurable.

Swadhyaya—*Self-Study*

Any activity that cultivates self-reflective consciousness can be considered *swadhyaya*. The soul tends to be lured by those activities that will best illuminate it. Because people are so different in their proclivities, one person may be drawn to write, while another will discover herself through painting or athletics. Another person may come to know himself through mastering an instrument, or through service at a hospice. Still another may learn hidden aspects of herself through the practice of meditation. The form that this self-study takes is inconsequential. Whatever the practice, as long as there is an intention to know yourself through it, and the commitment to see the process through, almost any activity can become an opportunity for learning about yourself. *Swadhyaya* means staying with our process through thick and thin because it's usually when the going gets rough that we have the greatest opportunity to learn about ourselves.

While self-study uncovers our strengths, authentic *swadhyaya* also ruthlessly uncovers our weakness, foibles, addictions, habit patterns, and negative tendencies. This isn't always the most cheering news. The worst thing we can do at these times is give ourselves the double whammy of both uncovering a soft spot and beating ourselves up for what we perceive as a fatal flaw. At these times, it's important actually to welcome and accept our limitations. When we welcome a limitation, we can get close enough to ourselves to see the roots of our anger, impatience, or self-loathing. We can have a little compassion for the forces and conditions that molded our behaviors and beliefs, and in so doing develop more skill in handling, containing, and redirecting previously self-destructive tendencies. The degree to which we can do this for ourselves is the degree to which we will be tolerant of other people's weaknesses and flaws. Self-study is a big task.

Self-study also can become psychically incestuous when the same self that may be confused and fragmented attempts to see itself. This is why it can be so helpful (not to mention expedient) to secure the help of a mentor, teacher, or close friend to support your self-study. If you've ever said that someone "just doesn't see himself" and watched him enact the same self-destructive behaviors again and again, just consider how likely it is that you too are blind to your own faults. A skillful mentor, and that can be anyone from a wise aunt to a therapist to a bona fide guru, can find loving ways to help you see yourself as you really are.

Ishvarapranidhana—*Celebration of the Spiritual*

Life is not inherently meaningful. We *make* meaning happen through the attention and care we express through our actions. We make meaning happen when we set a table with care, when we light a candle before practicing, or when we remove our shoes before entering a temple. Yoga tells us that the spiritual suffuses everything— it is simply that we are too busy, too distracted, or too insensitive to notice the extraordinary omnipresence that dwells in all things. So one of the first ways that we can practice *ishvarapranidhana* is by putting aside some time each day, even a few minutes, to avail ourselves of an intelligence larger than our own. This might take the form of communing with your garden at dawn, taking a few moments on the bus to breathe slowly and clear your mind, or engaging in a more formal practice such as a daily reading, prayer, ritual, or meditation. This practice requires that we have recognized that there is some omnipresent force larger than ourselves that is guiding and directing the course of our lives. We all have had the experience of looking back at some event in our life that at the time may have seemed painful, confusing and disruptive, but later, in retrospect, made perfect sense in the context of our personal destiny. We recognize that the change that occurred during that time was necessary for our growth, and that we are happier for it. The catch is that it's hard to see the bigger picture when you think you are the great controller of your life. When you are the great controller, you fail to recognize that supposed coincidences, accidents, and chance meetings all have some greater significance in the larger scheme of your destiny. When you are the master of your universe, it's hard to trust anything but your own self-made plans. When we don't have this recognition that there's a bigger story going on, we get caught up in our personal drama and a frustrating cycle of resistance to change. *Ishvarapranidhana* asks us to go quietly, even when it's not possible to see exactly where things are headed. At first this can be frightening, like being suspended in the air between one trapeze bar and another, but, over time, this not knowing exactly how life is going to unfold and the giving up of our frantic attempts to manipulate and control makes each day an adventure. It makes our life a horse race right up until the very finish!

Ultimately, *ishvarapranidhana* means surrendering our personal will to this intelligence so we can fulfill our destiny. The first step in this practice is attuning ourselves to perceive a larger perspective. By setting aside enough time to get quiet and clear, we can begin to differentiate between the cluttered thoughts of our ordinary mind and the resonant intelligence that comes through as intuition. Rather than trying to unravel the mystery, we start to embody the mystery of life. When we embody the mystery, we begin to experience meaning where before we experienced numbness. When we drink a glass of water, we taste it; when a cool breeze brushes our bare skin, we feel it; and when a stranger speaks to us, we listen. Everything and anything can become a sign of this intelligence.

Eventually we are spontaneously drawn to look at the purpose of our life with a new eye. One starts to ask, How can my life be useful to others? Living the answer is neither spiritual insurance nor a guarantee against hardship, but it is insurance against living a meaningless life, a life that at its end we regret.

WHAT ARE YOGA *ASANAS* AND WHY PRACTICE THEM?

Given the central importance of the *yamas* and *niyamas,* one might wonder why it would be necessary to practice the other limbs of yoga. Would it not be enough to be compassionate, truthful, and content? Why would it be important to take the time to stretch our backs or to listen to our breath? If not for the tremendous importance of grounding spirituality in the body, it's unlikely that the great sages would have listed *asana* practice as the second limb. This is why I have chosen to focus in such detail on this dimension of practice. What is *asana* practice all about?

The word *asana* is usually translated as "pose" or "posture," but its more literal meaning is "comfortable seat." Through their observations of nature, the yogis discovered a vast repertoire of energetic expressions, each of which had not only a strong physical effect on the body but also a concomitant psychological effect. Each movement demands that we hone some aspect of our consciousness and use ourselves in a new way. The vast diversity of *asanas* is no accident, for through exploring both familiar and unfamiliar postures we are also expanding our consciousness, so that regardless of the situation or form we find ourselves in, we can remain "comfortably seated" in our center. Intrinsic to this practice is the uncompromising belief that every aspect of the body is pervaded by consciousness. *Asana* practice is a way to develop this interior awareness.

While a dancer's or athlete's internal impulses result in movement that takes him into space, in *asana* practice our internal impulses are contained inside the dynamic form of the posture. When you witness a yoga practitioner skilled in this dynamic internal dance, you have the sense that the body is in continuous subtle motion. What distinguishes an *asana* from a stretch or calisthenic exercise is that in *asana* practice we focus our mind's attention completely *in* the body so that we can move as a unified whole and so we can perceive what the body has to tell us. We don't do something *to* the body, we *become* the body. In the West we rarely do this. We watch TV while we stretch; we read a book while we climb the StairMaster; we think about our problems while we take a walk, all the time living a short distance from the body. So *asana* practice is a reunion between the usually separated body-mind.

Apart from the vibrant health, flexibility, and stamina this unified body-mind brings us, living in the body is also an integral aspect of spiritual practice. The most tangible way that we can know what it means to be compassionate or not grasping is directly through the cellular experience of the body. The most direct way that we can learn what it means to let go is through the body. When we have a self-destructive addiction—the impulse to overeat or to take drugs—this happens through the entrenchment of neurological and physiological patterns in our bodies. And on a more basic level, it's hard to feel focused and purposeful when our bodies are full of aches and pains or burdened with illness and disease.

While I have given the practice of *asanas* great emphasis in this book, it is not because the perfection of the body or of yoga postures is the goal of yoga practice. This down-to-earth, flesh-and-bones practice is simply one of the most direct and expedient ways to meet yourself. It is a good place to begin. Whether you meet yourself through standing on your feet or standing on your head is irrelevant. It's important, therefore, not to make the mistake of thinking that the perfection of the yoga *asanas* is the goal, or that you'll be good at yoga only once you've mastered the more difficult postures. The *asanas* are useful maps to explore yourself, but they are not the territory. The goal of *asana* practice is to live in your body and to learn to perceive clearly through it. If you can master the Four Noble Acts, as I like to call them, of sitting, standing, walking, and lying down with ease, you will have mastered the basics of living an embodied spiritual life. This book gives you the tools to do this and to go further if you wish.

The emphasis on *asana* practice is also specific to the age we live in, for we live in a time of extreme dissociation from bodily experience. When we are not in our bodies, we are dissociated from our instincts, intuitions, feelings and insights, and it becomes possible to dissociate ourselves from other people's feelings, and other people's suffering. The insidious ways in which we become numb to our bodily experience and the feelings and perceptions that arise from them leave us powerless to know who we are, what we believe in, and what kind of world we wish to create. If we do not know when we are breathing in and when we are breathing out, when we are unable to perceive gross levels of tension, how then can we possibly know how to create a balanced world? Every violent impulse begins in a body filled with tension; every failure to reach out to someone in need begins in a body that has forgotten how to feel. There has never been a back problem or a mental problem that didn't have a body attached to it. This limb of yoga practice reattaches us to our body. In reattaching ourselves to our bodies we reattach ourselves to the responsibility of living a life guided by the undeniable wisdom of our body.

PRACTICING WITH JOYFULNESS

When we begin practice, we may feel far from happy within ourselves. In fact, even the semblance of happiness may seem as remote to us as winning the lottery. We may feel utterly confused, buried in self-destructive habits, and encumbered by difficulties, whether emotional, physical, or material, that appear insurmountable. Our bodies may feel as stiff and knotted as an old tree, and our minds a jumble of worries and neuroses. Platitudes about the peace and happiness available to us right now sound empty in the face of our very real pain. Most of us begin like this, and even those who feel some sense of inner balance often find that underneath the thin veneer of appearances, there is much work to be done.

How do we go about doing this work without becoming discouraged by the enormity of the task? Unless we can find a way to practice with joyfulness, working with our difficulties rather than against them, practice will be an experience of frustration and disappointment. Unless we can find a way to enjoy what we are doing right now, yoga practice will become a negative time, and ultimately we'll develop a strong resistance even to stepping onto the mat.

A story may help you to understand what I mean. Many years ago I moved into a derelict house. The back door was nailed shut and had not been opened for fifteen years; once pried open it revealed a six-foot wall of seemingly impenetrable blackberry bushes, vines, and crabgrass. I wanted a garden. For many months I looked in despair through the window of the back door. The task seemed too large and too difficult. Then I decided upon a strategy that my mind could grasp. I decided that I would divide the project into four-foot increments. Every week I would clear a four-foot patch of garden. The backyard was sixty-five feet long! As I would begin to dig and root, cutting and pulling my tiny patch, I resolved that I would focus my attention only on the four-foot patch. I would not even look at the other sixty-one feet of garden left to clear. Within minutes of beginning I would become completely absorbed in the insects, the tiny plants uncovered, and the pleasure of digging my hands into the brown earth. Each four-foot patch took about three hours because the crabgrass had to be dug out completely and the earth was rock hard. But three hours a week was an easily manageable commitment. When I was finished with the patch, I would step back and admire my good work, never allowing myself to consider the chaotic mess left remaining. How wonderful it looked! Each four-foot patch was a unique wonder. Pathways buried two feet under emerged. A lawn mower, enveloped by grass (proof of the law of karma), was discovered. Not only was the task challenging, it became an adventure, and I eagerly anticipated what I might find each week. Within a year I had a beautiful lawn, an herb garden, and a patch of flowers to enjoy. But, more important, I enjoyed the process of transforming an inhospitable patch of ground into an urban paradise.

When you begin to practice, you may feel very bound in your body and mind, not unlike the densely woven crabgrass of my garden. You can choose to fight with yourself, pulling and tugging on yourself as a way to force your own metamorphosis. If you've ever encountered a weed with deep roots, you know the futility of pulling at the stem knowing full well some digging is in order! There's a moment when you can cheerfully accept the task and set to it with full vigor, or turn sour and miserable in the face of such work. There's a moment when you can resign yourself to the patient work ahead or give in to the impulse to pull on the stem before the ground has been dug deep enough. The first step is accepting that some deep work needs to be done and then deciding to make this a positive, uplifting experience.

In yoga practice you can do this by dividing your experience into incremental breaths and taking care of only that which arises in one breath cycle and no more. In this way almost any difficulty becomes manageable. Rather than focusing on how much further you wish you could go, or comparing your meager efforts with those of someone who is more adept, you can choose to focus on what you are accomplishing in each breath. Maybe today you open your hip five millimeters farther, or you manage to sit comfortably in meditation for the first time. As you investigate the tightness around your hip you discover ways to release it; as you sit for five more minutes you discover that those "urgent" matters were really not so urgent. It is only through these tiny, slow, and progressive openings that deep, profound change occurs. It is your choice to take pleasure in these small awakenings or to disregard your efforts as insignificant in the face of how much further you have to go. You can choose to have a sense of humor about your dilemma or fester in negativity. Whom would you like to garden with?

When we make practice a joyful time, it is also much more likely that we are growing more deeply within our spiritual life. When we get hooked into striving toward where we think we should be and how far we ought to be able to go, in truth we are somewhere else all the time. We are in our fantasy, our ideas, our concepts, and our judgments. There's not much room in there to perceive and appreciate what's actually happening. Even when we feel pain, even when we face great difficulty, we can take refuge in our practice. There will inevitably be times when progress is slow, when injury or illness or life circumstances limit our ability to do the outward forms. But this doesn't limit our ability to plumb the depths of our inner life.

Each day as you step onto your mat, make a decision to enjoy just where you are right now. Take a few moments, too, to contemplate how fortunate you are to be practicing this wonderful art. A casual glance at the morning paper is proof enough of the vast suffering, poverty, violence, and homelessness that is the lot of so many human beings. If you are standing on a yoga mat and have the time to practice even fifteen minutes, you are a fortunate person. If you have a yoga teacher, you have an invaluable gift and life tool available to very few people. In the spirit of this gratefulness, let your practice begin.

II

The Seven Moving Principles

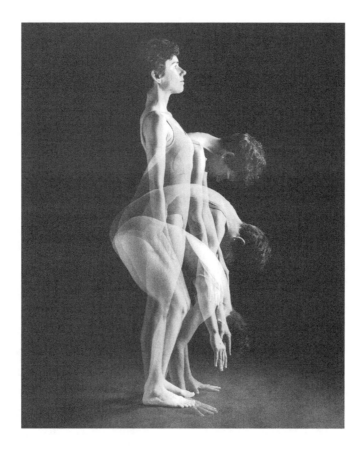

Introduction

*J*ust as there is an invisible force that produces the organic symmetry of a
towering pine's branches, the spiral vortex of an ocean wave, and the endless
cycle of days and nights that govern our lives, so, too, our human bodies are governed by intrinsically intelligent patterns. From the extraordinary moment when
egg and sperm are ignited into being, our bodies form a design unlike any other
that has ever been or will ever be through a wondrous process that is both a repli-
cation of an ancient blueprint and a uniquely individual expression. Our cells mul-
tiply and divide, expanding and differentiating into the specific expression that
makes us unique, condensing and disappearing back into this same matrix when
we die. The inner scaffolding of bones, the tensile fiber of muscles, the processing
organs, innervating nerves, and the oceanic fluid systems of the body are arranged
into the symphony we call the human body. But these structures alone do not
make a body. Just as a lightbulb is useless until it is connected to electricity, the raw
substance of our body does not become human until it is infused with the force of
life. This mysterious life force expresses itself through the projection of light from
our eyes; it circulates the blood through our hearts and causes the ceaseless cycle of
inspiration and expiration.

This life force also provides us with a blueprint for optimal movement in the
form of universal movement patterns that govern all our actions. These patterns

organize our intentions into effortless action. The patterns are biologically innate templates that are programmed into our bodies to permit us to move with ease and power. Some arise as if by an internal time clock, just as we might expect a baby to begin speaking by a certain month. Others happen through our desire to explore the world; the first push from a leg or reach of a fingertip taking us toward a beckoning father or colorful toy. They manifest as a series of overlapping and mutually dependent patterns, a language of movement that gives us kinesthetic fluency.

We see the underlying play of movement patterns all the time but are rarely aware of the content of what we see. We can identify a person with neurological disorders far in the distance because we are able to distinguish that the pattern of their gait is different from the normal pattern we have grown to recognize. The function of a symbol or pattern enables us to go beyond the limitation of seeing life as fragments and disparate parts and link these parts into a cohesive whole. While we could learn to walk by breaking down the activity into thousands of separate details, each of which are essential to succeed, this would be an impossibly difficult and frustrating way to go about the task. Rather, we learn to move through patterns.

Because the patterns are designed to create the most efficient pathways for movement and expression, once you have discovered how to engage their support you will be able to figure out the alignment of *any* posture by yourself. This will liberate you from dependence on a teacher, allowing you to trust and follow your own instinctual alignment process.

When you find the "knack" of a movement, you have unknowingly found the cohesive movement pattern that was needed to support your action. Because many of the patterns, like the movement of breathing, are governed by lower brain function, reawakening them involves using a different part of the mind than many of us are accustomed to engaging. Unfortunately, most of us have been taught movement in an overly intellectual, one-step-at-a-time way, with some yoga methodologies breaking down the yoga postures into a minutia of points and details. If you've ever tried to talk yourself up into a handstand by placing your shoulders and your wrists and your head—and so on—in exactly the right way, you know how frustrating this can be. It's like going to a filing cabinet for the information but opening up the wrong drawer. When we learn through patterns, we learn through a more sensate, felt, experiential mode of exploration and discovery. To do this we have to open the mind, becoming childlike so that the body can reveal to us the knowledge with which it was born.

At first glance through any comprehensive yoga text it is likely the reader will be overwhelmed by the sheer number and apparent complexity of the yoga *asanas* and practices. Yet, because human movement develops logically, we can simplify and at the same time deepen our understanding of these amazing practices by first learning and integrating the underlying movement principles that encompass all movement. This is not merely a physical or mechanical process. Each movement pattern and principle is directly related to an organizing pattern of consciousness. Thus, when you learn to breathe freely, you are also learning to think and live freely. When you learn a simple skill such as standing with ease, you learn about right relationship, trust, and the interconnectedness of all things.

Also, at first glance the yoga *asanas* may appear as static positions or postures, and why then would it be important to know about "moving" principles? When yoga was introduced to the West over a century ago, it was taught and adapted in a way that the objective Western mind could understand. While this objectification had the positive effect of planting the seeds of yoga in a new culture, some of the more profound and meaningful aspects of the practice have been lost or misunderstood. In large part what has been passed on and, unfortunately, continues to be propagated is the form of the practice without the living, vital contents. The yoga *asanas,* while appearing relatively static compared to other movements, are actually still dances swirling with internal motion. The form of each *asana* acts as a container for these subtle yet powerful internal movements. The untrained eye sees no visible movement, but on further investigation, an *asana* practiced in this vital way is easy to distinguish. When a dancer moves, his actions take him into space, and thus his energy tends to be dissipated by his efforts. In yoga we direct movement inside the body so that its positive effects serve to cleanse and regenerate us. The key to rediscovering the original life of the practices does not lie in contrived, artificial techniques that we impose on the body, but rather in listening to and following the laws of the natural world.

The following seven guiding movement principles are true for all movements. When you have explored each one, you will find that they carry through all your activities and act as a guiding thread for the entire repertoire of yoga practices. Practicing yoga without the support of these principles would be like trying to build a house without architectural plans. This foundation material will allow you to progress more quickly, and because this information comprises a series of keystones for unlocking the yoga *asanas,* if you do encounter difficulty, you will be able to trace your difficulty back to one or more of these principles.

To fully digest how each principle works, explore each for a few weeks before moving on to the next. Take your time. This preliminary work will stand you in good stead as you progress into the more specific applications later in the book. As you become more adept at the postures and begin a daily home practice, you can focus on one principle as a guiding theme for your entire practice. You may find that you have already integrated many of these principles into your life, while others may, at first, feel foreign and awkward. Knowing your strengths as well as your weaknesses will allow you to retrace your steps and find solutions to difficulties you encounter later.

THE PROCESS OF INQUIRY

The "inquiries" that are sprinkled throughout this book are distinctly different from the exercises so familiar to the Western mind. The word *exercise* usually implies some kind of repetitive activity (often unpleasant) that we will ourselves to do. "Doing an exercise" also assumes there is a set result we are trying to achieve, and the fore-knowledge of this "correct" result tends to color our perceptions of that which is expected of us. The purpose of the inquiries is to provide you with a situation in which you can explore and discover new skills for yourself. While it is likely you will discover some of the principles laid out in the following sections, it is also likely that by keeping your perceptual process open and entering each inquiry in a spirit of curiosity, you will discover information beyond that which I have suggested.

Everyone has her own style of learning, but here are a few suggestions for getting the most out of the inquiries. It is helpful first to visualize the aspect of the body you wish to make more tangible. By sensing and feeling the texture, weight, and quality of that part, you can continue your investigation using active imagination, touch, movement, and focused breathing. As you enter an inquiry the most important attitude to bring with you is one of inquisitiveness and open-mindedness. *If there is no ideal to the process of perception, then anything you feel or sense is worthy of your observation.* No movement, thought, or impulse is insignificant in open awareness. There is no good or bad perception. This nondiscriminatory awareness will allow you to go far beyond the limited perspective that is your lot when your sole concern is to "get it right." But mostly inquiries provide a relaxed atmosphere to learn without the fear of failure or the pressure of succeeding by deadline. Without these largely self-imposed pressures how delightful it is to play, experiment, and find anew the true delight of learning. Surely it was this same process of experimentation that allowed the ancient yogis to discover the vast and creative range of practices handed down to us today. It is only through a recapitulation of this process that we can discover the inner meaning of the practice and go beyond mechanical repetition.

PREPARING FOR YOUR PRACTICE

Before you begin your yoga practice take a refreshing shower or bath and change into loose-fitting clothes. It's a good idea to practice on an empty stomach, preferably after you have gone to the bathroom in the morning. Remove any restrictive clothing such as bras or belts and, whenever possible, turn off the sound to the phone, TV, or stereo. Close the door to your practice room, and make sure the room is warm and the floor well padded if you are lying down. If you don't live alone, let the rest of your household know you don't want to be disturbed for a while. Take the time to prepare yourself and your surroundings so you'll get the most out of each session.

CREATING A PRACTICE SPACE

Creating a sacred space is so essential to establishing a consistent practice that it is worth a note here. Reserving a space for practice and making it special in some way that distinguishes it from the rest of your everyday life is a concrete way of reinforcing to yourself and others around you the importance and meaning of your practice.

Whether you have the luxury of an extra room in your home or only a small corner in your bedroom or living room, make sure that the space you have selected is clean and free of dust and insects. Organize your yoga equipment (see page 27) neatly in this space so you do not have to interrupt your practice to find things. Ideally the space will have a hardwood floor or other firm surface and enough clear wall space so you can stand with your back to the wall and with your arms out-stretched.

Now, the most important part: Make this space special in some way. A small table, stool, or shelf, or a clear space on the wall can act as a central focus. Here are some possibilities:

- Light a candle or stick of incense when you practice.
- Place one fresh flower in a bud vase there daily.
- Make an arrangement of objects of significance. This could be as simple as a plain bowl filled with bright yellow lemons, or a collection of seashells, stones, or small statues of deities.
- Keep a small plant, and tend to it before you practice.
- Hang a picture of someone who has inspired you. If there are religious or spiritual teachers who are central to your life, give them a place in your practice space. If there are mentors or friends who have supported and helped you, their presence here may help you during times of difficulty.

Don't get carried away with too many objects, for you will want this space to be uncluttered. Removing stacks of books and household paraphernalia will prevent you from being distracted by everyday concerns. Each time you practice in this special place it grows in power such that others may even comment on the calm and peaceful feeling they have when they are in your special place. After a while the space itself may draw you there to do your practice, providing essential and necessary solace in the midst of life's challenges and pressures.

GETTING STARTED

Just as a runner needs a good pair of running shoes, you'll need some essential pieces of equipment, called yoga props, to get the most out of your practice. As your practice develops you may also wish to invest in other props or accessories that will give you greater versatility. Most are available at your local yoga studio or through yoga prop companies. Both *Yoga Journal* and *Yoga International* magazines have extensive listings for yoga prop companies as well as an annual listing of yoga teachers and centers throughout the world.

ESSENTIAL YOGA EQUIPMENT

- **A Yoga "Sticky" Mat** (1/8″ × 24″ × 68″): A yoga mat will prevent your feet, hands, and elbows from slipping on the floor and give your body cushioning and protection from cold floors.

- **Blankets:** You'll need three to four tightly woven blankets (preferably wool or high-quality cotton), big enough to cover your body from head to toe. Blankets can be folded, rolled, stacked, and rearranged in a thousand ways to adapt postures, and offer you cushioning and warmth as well. Avoid using quilts, bedspreads, and nylon blankets as these offer too little support. Your local army surplus store may be a good place to look for inexpensive practice blankets. Reserve these for yoga alone—cracker crumbs and dog hair do nothing to inspire a yoga practice!

- **A Tie** (1.5″ × 6′–8′): A strong bathrobe tie or leather belt will suffice in the beginning. Proper yoga ties are made of tightly woven cotton webbing and are finished with steel D-ring buckles or plastic cinch closures. A tie allows you to extend the length of your arm so you can modify poses for your ability level. They can also be used as traction devices and for securing your limbs in restorative postures.

- **A Block** (4″ × 6″ × 9″): A solid wooden block will allow you to support yourself in postures in which you might otherwise have to reach all the way to the floor. Yoga prop companies now make these in light, high-density foam, which makes them easy to move around and carry for travel. Hardcover books and telephone books make handy alternatives.

- **A Folding Chair:** Choose a chair that is sturdy, with nonslip feet. You can use the chair to modify difficult postures and for specific stretches.

YOGA ACCESSORIES

While they are not essential, many of these items will allow you to home in on difficult tight spots and refine your practice further. You will find most in any well-equipped yoga studio, where a teacher can show you how to use them safely.

- **Bolsters** (9″ × 9″ × 27″): A bolster is a cylindrical or rectangular densely packed cushion. These provide excellent support for many of the yoga postures in which you would otherwise have to stack many blankets. Thus, they save time! Also, as a beginner you may need substantial propping in some postures until your body becomes more flexible.

- **Eye Bags** ($1'' \times 4'' \times 8.5''$): Small silk- or cotton-covered pouches filled with flax seeds or plastic beads. These cover the eyes, blocking out light and distractions, and are fantastic aids for relaxation. Store eye bags in a sealed container because rodents love to eat the seeds! A dark-colored silk or cotton scarf makes a good alternative, especially when traveling.

- **Elastic Bandage** ($4'' \times 48''$): Athletic-type wrap bandages easily found in a drugstore. These can be gently wound around the head to induce deep relaxation.

- **Sandbags** ($2'' \times 7'' \times 17''$): Larger rectangular bags made from densely woven fabric such as denim, canvas, or corduroy and filled with ten pounds of sterilized sand. Sandbags can be used to anchor a part of the body or provide deep pressure that might otherwise have been provided by a teacher's adjustment. If you make your own, fill them only three-quarters of the way full so they are not too stiff or blocky and will conform to the shape of your body. Bags of beans or rice make good alternatives.

- **Gymnic Balls:** These large plastic balls come in sizes from 16 to 37 inches in diameter and are mostly used for releasing the back, belly, and shoulders into extension. Generally speaking, the larger the ball the easier back-bending will be, with smaller balls offering more intense opening to specific areas of the back. They also make excellent chairs for home or office use. At our yoga studio our students love to use the balls as soon as they enter class, to counter the effects of a long day of sitting at the office.

- **Wrist Wedges:** The prevalence of overuse syndromes and carpal tunnel injuries has increased enormously since the advent of word processing. Many people who have problems with their wrists and arms will find a wrist wedge an invaluable aid in those poses where the wrist is extended and bearing weight. A wrist wedge raises the lower palm to decrease the angle of extension. Although wrist wedges are usually made of high-density foam, my preference is for students to use a wooden slant board because this provides the best support for the wrist joint. You can make a slant board with a ¾-inch-thick piece of lumber, approximately 10 inches wide by 2 feet long. Glue a piece of sticky mat all the way around the board. Use a second mat rolled into a cylinder and place underneath one side of the board. The palms of your hands will be on the board while your fingers will be on the floor. As your wrists heal and become more agile, you can gradually reduce the diameter of the cylinder, thereby reducing the angle of the slant.

THE SEVEN MOVING PRINCIPLES

1. BREATHE
   Let the Breath Move You

2. YIELD
   Yield to the Earth: Weight and Levity

3. RADIATE
   Move from the Inside Out: The Human Starfish

4. CENTER
   Maintain the Integrity of the Spine: The Central Axis

5. SUPPORT
   Establish Foundations of Support: Structural Building Blocks

6. ALIGN
   Create Clear Lines of Force: Alignment and Sequential Flow

7. ENGAGE
   Engage the Whole Body: The Democratic Body Community

RETURN
   Return the Mind to Original Silence: Developing Clear Perception

1. Breathe
Let the Breath Move You

*The breath arises out of stillness, expands, condenses, and returns to
this ground of stillness. Oscillation is an intrinsic part of life and all movements.*

The First Movement

From the moment of conception our bodies begin to breathe. Each cell in the body expands, condenses, and rests in an internal rhythmic pattern, a pattern that will become amplified into full-body breathing at the moment of birth. This first movement is the basic template for our existence. Whether we are sitting still, running up a hill, or sound asleep, the breath acts as a continuous resonant presence infusing and influencing all other processes, from the chemical reactions of our cells to our moment-to-moment psychological and emotional state.

The fundamental nature of the breath is that it is in a constant state of oscillation. Just as the tides ebb and flow, we breathe in and out in an ongoing rhythm

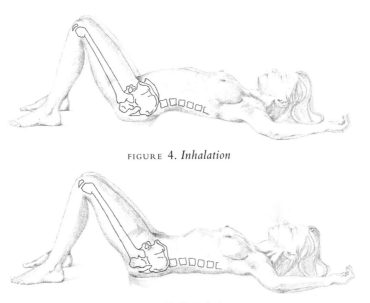

FIGURE 4. *Inhalation*

FIGURE 5. *Exhalation*

4 & 5. Pelvic and Spinal Oscillation: When you breathe, the pelvis rocks slightly, causing the entire spine to change shape. As you inhale, the abdomen swells, causing the pelvis to rock forward and the lumbar spine to arch. As you exhale, the abdomen condenses, causing the pelvis to rock back, and under which flattens and elongates the lumbar spine.

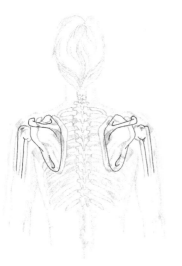

FIGURE 6

6. Shoulder Oscillation: When you breathe in, the ribs expand up and out, causing the shoulder blades to migrate away from the spine. The arm bones go along for the ride, expanding outward with the inhalation. As you breathe out, the ribs move down and back, and both the arms and shoulder blades retract back to their original position.

that ceases only when we take our last breath. All other physical and psychological patterns build successively from this one central motif (Figures 4, 5, and 6). For this reason, if the movement of the breath is restricted or distorted in some way, all other patterns of our movement and consciousness will also be restricted or distorted. Every other process in the body community is reliant upon this one central process.

The oscillation of breathing is a perfect mirror of the fluctuations of life. Life is like a swinging pendulum, some changes bringing with them difficulties and pain and other changes bringing with them ease and joy. If we are open to this process, life *will* move us. If we are unable to integrate life's changes, we begin to resist by restricting our breath. When we hold the breath and try to control life or stop changes from happening, we are saying that we do not want to be moved. In those moments our desire for certainty has become much stronger than our desire to be dynamically alive. Breathing freely is a courageous act. What we discover is that our desire for stasis, our clinging to the life we know, and our bending of every situation to the security of our mental constructs are the very things that destroy our creativity and ability to live freely.

Breathing *happens* to us when we remove the obstacles we have erected to its free movement. As such, the most common misunderstanding about breathing is that it improves through a forceful effort of the will. Anyone who has tried to breathe deeper through aggressive strategies knows that mechanical efforts to breathe better only result in making the breathing more restricted and more limited.

Breathing is both a process that happens unconsciously or automatically and a process that can be controlled consciously through the will of our minds. At one end of a continuum breathing remains unconscious so that we can go about our business without having constantly to think about taking a breath in or out. At the other end of the continuum breathing can be controlled and manipulated. The yogis developed sophisticated protocols for unleashing the power of the breath, called *pranayama* practices. The root word *pra* denotes constancy, and *na* means movement.[1]

Therefore prana is a force in constant motion. In between these two ends of the continuum lies a third possibility, one that should precede any formal *pranayama* practice, and that is the place where we simply become conscious of being breathed. We allow this essential breathing to happen to us naturally.

Becoming attuned to your breath is like learning to dance the waltz with another person. At first you have to become familiar with your dance partner—how he moves, when he moves, and where he moves. To be a good dance partner with the breath you must be suggestible and let the wisdom of the breath guide *all* of your movements. As you learn to follow the lead of the breath, you will know what to do next. I call this "moving inside the breath." At other times, when you do not have a connection to your breath, you are moving "outside" the breath. When you do this, it will feel like dancing the waltz by yourself. As you become more masterfully attuned to your breath, the division between leader and follower dissolves and all that is left is the dance itself.

～ INQUIRY ～

Letting the Breath Move You

You can do this inquiry in almost any position: lying on your back, side, or belly; sitting or standing; or in any yoga *asana* or activity. The two positions I have chosen, however, allow you to feel oscillation very clearly. As you begin to sense the nature of the oscillating breath, I encourage you to continue exploring the work in different positions, for each reveals new information.

Stand with your feet hips-width apart. Bend your knees generously and allow your spine to fold forward over your legs (Figures 7 and 8). Let the head, neck, and the arms drape. If this position is uncomfortable because of the tightness along the back of your legs or in your spine, you can fold forward sitting in a chair with your feet wide apart. In this variation your head will hang between your legs and your arms will drape along the outside of your knees.

Let go of any agenda concerning how far you stretch forward. Then begin to sense and feel your breath entering and leaving your body. Feel the way the breathing expands and condenses the whole body. Notice that there are brief moments in between the expanding and condensing during which the body and the breath are still. These pauses are rather like the pause of the pendulum when it reaches its arc in space before continuing its trajectory to the other side.

From stillness the breath expands and moves you, and as it condenses it moves you, returning back to the ground of stillness before beginning the cycle again. Imagine your bones are like tiny, light boats bobbing up and down on the current of your breathing. As you give yourself over to this current you find that your body becomes married to the breath. A thousand tiny shifts, rotations, openings, and closings are happening throughout the entire body. Let yourself "be breathed."

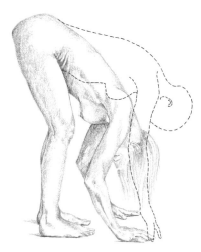

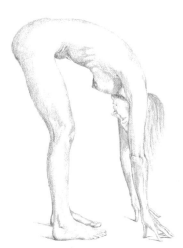

FIGURE 7

FIGURE 8. *Incorrect*

7 & 8. Full Body Oscillation: Whether in a simple movement like this or in a yoga posture, the body is continually expanding and condensing in synchrony with the breath. If you attempt to hold your body in a set position as shown in Figure 8 you will restrict the free movement of breath throughout your body.

Then begin to sense and feel more acutely exactly *how* you are being moved. Can you feel your spine being alternately lifted and lowered? Can you feel your shoulder blades shifting position? Can you feel your spine changing shape, and if so, how does it change shape when you breathe in and out? Are your arms a part of this movement, or do they feel cut off from the central current of the breath? Do your head and neck pulse slightly, nodding up and down with the incoming and outgoing breath? Where do you feel your body in *coparticipation* with the breath, and where do you feel cut off from its influence?

Your body's natural coparticipation with the breath happens when you stop controlling with your will and become *willing* to be moved. Opening your mouth, relaxing your jaw, and taking a few deep sighs as you breathe out through the mouth may help you to release tension and give yourself over to the process.

When you are ready, slowly curl up through your spine, supporting your back by placing your hands on your knees if necessary. As you come up to standing or sitting (if you did the exercise on a chair), take a moment to feel how the breath is continuing to move you.

> *Whatever movement or yoga* asana *you are practicing, allow the basic expanding, condensing pattern of the breath to express itself through you at all times. Then all your practice will become like a dance in which the invisible partner of the breath guides you.*

The illustrations that accompany these inquiries show some of the oscillations that occur in the body during breathing. Do you feel oscillation in these areas? It is difficult to show the nature of movement in a two-dimensional drawing, and quite impossible to reveal the infinite variety of movements caused by breathing. These illustrations are only a guide to spark your own further explorations. For a more in-depth discussion on breathing, see *The Breathing Book*, by Donna Farhi.

Amplifying the Breath

This inquiry is to help you to feel more clearly the marriage between breathing and movement. Begin by sitting comfortably in a chair. Place your hands on your thighs with your palms facing upward; gently stretch the hands so the fingers are softly extended but not tense. Then relax the hands and let the fingers curl inward so your palms form a slight hollow. In this way continue rhythmically to fold and unfold the hands for several minutes. Then begin to observe your breath. Do you notice any relationship between the movement of your hands and when you inhale and exhale?

Now extend this movement so that you open and turn out your arms and then relax and turn your arms inward. Let the movement expand into your chest so that your chest opens as you gently extend the arms and so that it settles and folds inward as you turn the arms inward. Let your entire spine come into the movement so that the whole body opens and closes like a sea anemone. Observe again how your breath is moving in response to the movement of the body. Let the movement get large and expansive. Feel how the breath changes as the movements grow larger, and then gradually over a period of minutes let the movements become smaller and smaller until you are quiet and still. As you cease the larger physical movements of the body and become quiet, can you still feel the echo of the movement inside you like a light alternately glowing and dimming?

This inquiry is an excellent and simple way to "kick-start" your breathing if it has become shallow or restricted. Even in the most public of places, opening and closing your hands will not draw attention to you. You can utilize it in a variety of forms during *asana* practice by slowly exaggerating folding and unfolding movements in any part of your body and gradually returning to relative stillness, listening and allowing the echo of the breath to continue.

Guiding the Breath: *Ujjayi*

The steps toward integration of body, mind, and breath can be compared to the apprenticeship of a sailor. Before a sailor can guide his boat he must know the nature of wind and water—their characteristics, rhythms, and cycles. Without a knowledge of these natural forces the most advanced and expensive boat in the world would be of little use. Once familiar with wind and water, the sailor can raise the sails and skillfully guide the boat where he wishes to go. No matter how masterful he is, however, he still cannot control the wind and water—he can only harness them.

When you have established a felt sense of your breathing and you are allowing it to move you freely, you are ready to move to the next stage of mastery—guiding the breath. Instead of canvas and spinnakers you have the natural opening of your throat and sail-like folds of your vocal cords. Called *ujjayi,* or the powerful breath, this basic *pranayama* technique involves a very slight closure of the vocal cords, or glottis, at the base of the throat. When done sensitively, your breathing will sound like the echo of the ocean inside a seashell—a deep but soft "sssss" on inhalation and "hmmmm" on exhalation. With *ujjayi* you can guide breath into the body in a fine, even spray that is deeply soothing to both the lungs and nervous system. The sound of *ujjayi* gives the mind a more tangible way to adhere to the breath's movements. With *ujjayi* you can spread the breath and direct it so that it permeates every cell of the body. All of the principles of moving with the breath still apply, only now you are guiding and refining these movements of the breath for your own benefit.

My experience with *ujjayi* is that it begins to happen naturally during the practice of *asanas,* and should never be forced or done so loudly that someone across the room can hear it. If you have a tendency to hold your breath and are only just beginning to feel your body moving in synchrony with your breath, I suggest you leave *ujjayi* alone. If you attempt to practice it too soon you will only be overlaying *ujjayi* upon your preexisting tension patterns and breath-holding habits. Take the time to explore the previous inquiries until you feel connected to your natural breath.

～ INQUIRY ～

Guiding the Breath

Practice a simple posture that you know already, or if you are new to yoga, try this inquiry in your chair. First, connect with the natural rhythm of your inhalation and exhalation and the movements in your body that correspond to these two phases of the breath. Then begin to practice *ujjayi,* feeling how this slight closure of your vocal cords allows you to modulate the volume, quality, and direction of the breath, much like using a nozzle on the end of a garden hose. Notice any changes in how you experience the posture. See the form of the posture in your mind's eye, and direct the breath so that it is moving in synchrony with the natural lines of the movement. Then, more specifically, guide the breath into any areas that feel resistant, tight, or dull, letting the spraylike quality of *ujjayi* penetrate each and every cell. At *any* time in your practice you can let go of *ujjayi* and return to normal breathing. Take a moment as you complete the posture to notice the effect this breathing practice has had on your state of mind.

The Principle in Practice
  - ～ Take time to connect with your breath *before* you begin a movement and then as you practice the *asana* go slowly enough so that you don't lose the connection.

～ Whenever you notice yourself holding your breath, exhale completely, blowing the air out through your mouth until the last whisper of air leaves your lungs. Wait for the inhalation to begin spontaneously, and then begin the yoga *asana* again with the support of your breath.

～ Slow down! Roughness, unevenness, or shortness of breath are signs that you are forcing the body to open too quickly or are moving in a way that is creating disharmony.

2. Yield
Yield to the Earth: Weight and Levity

Any surface of the body that makes contact with the ground must yield to the earth. Actively yielding to the earth creates a rebounding force away from the earth, elongating the body upward into space. Whenever the relationship of yielding to the earth is lost, breathing is restricted.

Our breathing does not take place as a discrete event separate from our environment. To be human involves standing upright, in relationship to the earth and to gravity. Thus, how we physically organize ourselves in relationship to these forces determines whether we breathe well or not. How we breathe, and why we may be holding our breath, can be understood in the context of three patterns:

Collapsing
Propping
Yielding

Collapsing (Figure 9): Most of us begin yoga from a state of collapse. In the collapsing pattern, we drop into the earth without the ability to use gravity to our advantage. As our structure sinks into the ground, we are unable to be a mediator between earth and heaven. This is the pattern of self-negation and results in (or is caused by) a lethargic, labored, and shallow breathing pattern.

Yielding (Figure 10): In between these two patterns is the posture of right relationship—yielding. Yielding happens when we allow the surfaces that are in contact with the earth to give their weight to the earth. At the same time we maintain enough integrity through our structure that we receive the rebound of gravity up through our bodies. If you have ever admired the graceful ease of tribal people as they stand and walk, you are seeing the result of this right relationship of the human being to the earth and sky. Similarly when you see a skilled dancer plié into the ground followed by a spectacular leap upward, you are seeing how the paradoxical giving of weight creates the conditions for levity.

The interesting thing about yielding is that it creates a "push" back through the body. This pushing action is different from propping because there is an ongoing alternation between yielding and pushing that is in synchrony with the breath—yield becomes push becomes yield. This dynamic pattern allows for an unimpeded flow of fluid circulation in the body and underlies ease and effortlessness in breathing at all times.

Propping (Figure 11): From the pattern of collapse we may attempt to pull ourselves up in a well-intentioned effort to stand up straight. We usually do this by actively pushing the earth away. This "push and push" pattern causes us to tighten our knees, lift the chest and shoulders, and thrust the spine forward. It is a posturing often encouraged by our parents and physical educators, and one that can be maintained only through willpower and vigilant attention. Not surprisingly, it is a very tiring posture to maintain because it is not self-renewing.

In this posture we are actually lifting ourselves away from the earth, as if to negate our relationship to it. Unconsciously we are saying that we do not trust the earth to hold us up. We create a chest-breathing pattern in which the secondary respiratory muscles high up in the body become overworked and uncomfortably tense. This type of breathing stimulates (or can be caused by) a fight-or-flight stress reaction.

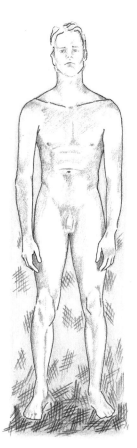

9. *Collapsing*

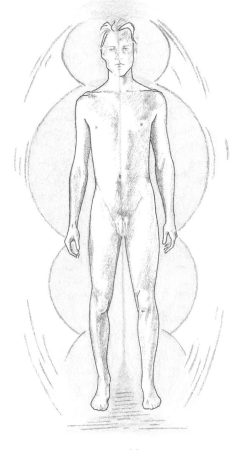

10. *Yielding*

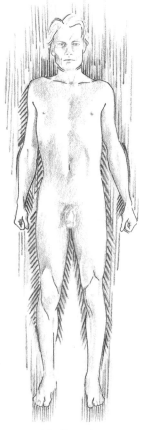

11. *Propping*

∼ INQUIRY ∼

Yielding to the Earth

Stand for a moment in your habitual way and observe the nature of your breathing. Then gradually let your weight collapse into the earth as if you had no bones. Feel all parts of your body sink into the earth. Observe the quality of your breathing now and the mind-state that accompanies this stance.

Now begin to push the earth away, continuously maintaining this pushing action. Tighten and lift up through your leg muscles. Draw your abdomen in, tighten your buttocks, and lift your chest and spine up against gravity. As you "prop" the body notice the quality of your breathing and the mind-state that accompanies this stance.

Finally, try the yielding pattern that exists in the middle of the continuum between propping and collapsing. From your propped stance slowly feel the weight of your leg bones feeding into the earth as you exhale. You might imagine the abdomen as an hourglass filled with sand. Keep the container of the hourglass lightly lifted as you pour the contents down through the center of your legs. Give the weight of your lower body into the earth and wait for the effortless rebound that will lift your body upward. You'll find that too little tone in your body will make you a poor conducting rod for the rebounding force, and too much tone and effort will prevent gravity and the earth from supporting you. Feel how you breathe when you prop or collapse, and notice how you breathe when you yield. What is the quality of your mind-state in yielding?

Yielding can be practiced whether standing, sitting, lying down, or being in motion, and of course, in all *asana* practice. Whatever surface touches the ground becomes the yielding surface, while all the parts of the body that are exposed to space expand into space.

The Principle in Practice

∼ Bending your knees when standing makes it easier to feel the action of yielding to the earth. You can fold and unfold any joint as a way to stimulate yielding. As you gradually straighten the limb, maintain the connection to the ground.

∼ Yield on your exhalation, feel the levity of the rebounding action on the inhalation.

∼ Tension in the toes, feet, ankles, knees, hips, and buttock area prevent yielding. Check these areas often.

3. Radiate

Move from the Inside Out: The Human Starfish

The six limbs of the body (head, tail, arms, and legs) connect to one another through the core of the body. The initiation of movement from the core to the limbs and from the limbs back to the core is called "navel radiation."[2]

Just as the starfish radiates outward with its sensitive extremities extending and feeding back into its central mouth, we too began in our mother's womb as a fetus receiving our nourishment and eliminating our waste through the umbilicus attached at our navel. The pattern of navel radiation sets up an energetic template for inner alignment between the core and the limbs. In this pattern, movement is initiated from the belly center and radiates out to any one or combination of the six limbs: head, tail, arms, or legs. In reverse the limbs can be drawn back to the center through the drawing action of the navel. Movement flows in undulatory waves from the center to the periphery and back again, amplifying an earlier template movement pattern—the expanding/condensing motion of breathing (Figure 12).

Navel radiation begins in utero and continues into early infancy. This pattern establishes the fluid energetic connections within our body to prepare us for the connections we will need to make later between the bones of our skeleton (Figure 13). As you can see from the illustrations, the fluidic template set up by navel radiation uses the same pathways we will need to link up when we connect our axial skeleton (the bones of the head, spine, and pelvis) and the appendicular skeleton (the bones of the arms and legs). The pattern continues to express itself in us as adults as an underlying energetic connection that provides cohesion between the parts of the body and the whole. When you engage the support of this pattern, aligning the body becomes an instinctual process.

To awaken this energetic connection there are three conditions that must be present. You can use these conditions as a three-step process to guide you into any *asana*.

Three Steps to Mastery

1. Establish a mobile, breathing core.
2. Connect the mobile core to the periphery.
3. Allow yourself to be moved.

1. Establish a mobile, breathing core: Simply ask yourself, "Am I breathing? Am I allowing my breath to move my central body? Is my core soft and mobile?" If your core is mobile, your belly, your entire spinal column, and all your internal organs will undulate with every breath. If the abdomen is hard and tight, or consciously held in, impulses cannot arise from the core or be received from the limbs back into the core. A tight belly is like a crashed car in the middle of an intersection—nothing can flow

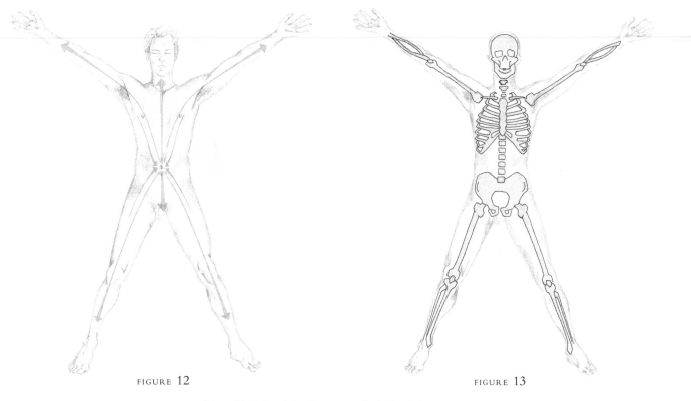

FIGURE 12   FIGURE 13

12 & 13. *Navel Radiation and Skeletal Structure*

through it until the obstruction is removed. Whenever you feel your abdomen tighten, place your hands there and breathe softly. Exhale and release.

2. Connect the mobile core to the periphery: Beginning from awareness of your mobile core, find a harmonious relationship between the core and each of your six limbs—head, tail (coccyx), arms, and legs. First find the energetic pathway between your core and your head and tail, and then find the link between your core and your arms and legs. All movement should connect smoothly from your core to your limbs and back again, and all your appendages should communicate with one another through the core. In any *asana,* your alignment is an attempt to find an energetic continuity throughout the body, bringing all parts into play as one whole. If you can find clear pathways connecting your core and your limbs, your breath will move unimpeded from your center out, and then draw back in again.

3. Allow yourself to be moved: Within the configuration in which you find yourself, can you allow yourself to be moved and changed by your breath? Let your pose be a "soft intention"—an open question rather than a definitive answer. As you move toward mastery in an *asana,* relinquish your attachment to being the *mover* of the posture; instead, let yourself *be moved.* Then there is no one left to do the posture, only the posture living itself through you.

Go slowly as you work through each step of this process. A mobile core is a source of enormous power and vitality, but you can tap into this source only through direct experience. In other words, striving to look as if you have an open center may give you the *appearance,* but never the true *experience,* of a mobile, breathing core. Let yourself experiment: make mistakes, fall over, and take as much time as you need. Whether you attain any particular pose becomes irrelevant once you make a commitment to honor and respect where you really are. When you practice with such honesty, your progress to physical mastery becomes a process that constantly brings you back to your true self.

～ INQUIRY ～

The Starfish

Lie on your belly on a soft surface, such as a carpeted floor or on folded blankets, allowing your head to turn to one side and your limbs to rest in any way that is comfortable. If turning your head is awkward, support your torso from the top of the breastbone to your public bone with a bolster, pillow, or stack of folded blankets so that your chest is elevated, with your head resting lightly on the ground (see Figure 230, page 239).

Allow yourself to release your weight into the earth, feeling the tremendous comfort and ease of embracing the earth with your soft front body. Take some time to let yourself settle and to connect with your breathing. Most important, don't try to make impressive movements, and resist the temptation to direct your body's movement mechanically. As you connect with your breathing, feel how the impulse of your breathing alternately expands and condenses, with the belly as the central mover. As you let your attention move to your belly, notice any impulses that begin from the belly and where these impulses travel. You may feel a wave moving from deep in the belly up the spine into the head or down into your tail. You might notice a ripple from your navel traveling into one hip and leg, or into a shoulder and arm on one side. As you feel these impulses, allow yourself to *coparticipate* with the movement. Rather than directing the movement by thinking and controlling, open yourself to feeling, and allow yourself to move spontaneously. Imagine your body as soft and boneless, able to ripple, slither, and undulate. Because everyone has her own style of moving (just as everyone walks differently), don't worry about doing the movement in a certain way.

Sustain a trace image of yourself as the human starfish, with your central intelligence at the level of your navel, and your sensitive limbs radiating out from there.

Begin to explore, expanding the limbs (either individually or in combination) away from the belly, as well as condensing, or feeding, the limbs back into the belly. As you condense, allow your belly to initiate the movement, as if the limbs were attached to it by invisible energetic strings being wound and unwound from a central spool. Feel free to roll onto your back or side, and to change levels as you play with all the possibilities. And whenever you tire, allow yourself to return to rest. Alternate these periods of deep, silent rest with activity until your inquiry is completed.

∿ INQUIRY ∿

Navel Radiation in Asanas

Every *asana*, regardless of its complexity, has as its foundation the pattern of navel radiation. Sometimes the linear and mechanical way in which we enter an *asana* belies the organic nature of the movement, or when we are showered with segmented and disparate instructions, our mind jumps from detail to detail without comprehending the matrix that holds the details so beautifully together. Or by "holding the pose" we deaden our own internal impulses. Take a moment to experiment with a few *asanas* that you know and to visualize the dynamic internal connections established by navel radiation. If you are new to yoga practice, try this inquiry in a simple standing position. Mentally draw the internal lines of force inside the position. Explore the posture as an expression of navel radiation, searching for the inner alignment that allows you to feel each limb in intimate connection to the center. When you practice in this way, you will feel the posture as a whole body expression. Be careful not to "set" your position as soon as you enter the *asana*. Enter the pose like a blind person finding her way through an unknown room. Once you do find a position that feels balanced, continue to remain "suggestible" and open to change.

The Principle in Practice

∿ *Always* begin by checking that your core is mobile and free.

∿ Initiate your movements from the center, like a flower blossoming. First find the connection between the navel and the head, and then work on the connection of the arms and legs to the core.

∿ Practice without arms. One of the most common errors in *asana* practice is to extend the limbs around a tight, unmoving core. If you tend to hold your belly in, try practicing without the use of your arms. Relax your arms by your sides and then place one hand firmly on your abdomen to help encourage more openness through your center. Use your hand to encourage the belly to open, then try extending your arms once again from this now mobile center.

4. Center

Maintain the Integrity of the Spine: The Central Axis

The integrity of the spinal column must be maintained in all movements. The spine elongates through the combined forces of gravity, the breath, and our directed intention.

Spinal Curves

The spinal column is a sensuously curved central axis through which gravity must fall straight and true. These two conditions may seem contradictory, but it is only when the spinal column contains harmonious curves that it can move freely and function to support other structures of the body with the *help* of gravity.

When we are still inside our mother's womb curled securely in the fetal position, the first two curvatures of the spine develop—the outwardly curved thoracic or upper back curve and the outwardly curved sacral area. These are called the *primary* curves of the spine. The twelve thoracic vertebrae are girded by the rib cage, while the five fused sacral vertebrae are firmly embedded in between the two sides of the pelvis. Because the shape of the bones in the thoracic and sacral spine, together with the stabilizing factor of the structures that connect to them, limits many movements, these two areas of the back tend to be more rigid and therefore more stable.

After we are born we begin to lift the head, fueled by our desire to see and experience the world beyond the ground. As we do so the bones of the neck curve inward to create the convex curvature of the cervical spine. To see farther beyond our immediate surroundings we prop ourselves up on our elbows, extending the lower back, and gradually, as we come to standing, the inward-moving curve of the lumbar spine develops. These two inwardly moving curves are called the *secondary curves* of the spine. The shape of the lumbar and cervical vertebrae and the angle of the articulating joints support movement in almost every plane. The extraordinary flexibility afforded by their structure makes these two areas of the back the most mobile. With mobility comes instability, so it

14. *Spinal Curves*

should not come as any surprise that the neck and lower back tend to be the most prone to problems and injury (Figure 14).

Apart from the shock-absorbing capacity of a curved structure, why should the spine be curved rather than straight? To understand this, we have to look at the spine's relationship to the rest of the body and to gravity. The two inward-moving curves in the lumbar and cervical spine provide support for the structures above them. As the lumbar vertebrae move inward they stack up underneath the rib cage and chest. In the same way, the cervical vertebrae move deep into the neck to provide a more central support for the head. As gravity passes through the crown of the head, it moves through the curve of the cervical and lumbar vertebrae, through the pelvis, and so on down to the feet. If the bones were not balanced over one another in this way, the muscles would be in a constant state of tension as they attempted to prevent the skeleton from collapsing under the downward pull of gravity. As we have seen in the inquiry on "Yielding to the Earth," the downward movement of gravity creates the conditions for the effortless rebound through the spine, a rebound that can occur only if the spine is an effective conduit. If one curve should become too deep, as in *hyperlordosis* (swayback), or too pronounced, as in *kyphosis* (rounded hunchback), or too flat, as in *hypolordosis* (which commonly occurs in both the lumbar and cervical spine), the spine becomes a less effective conduit for force. All of this said, there is no one ideal spinal shape. Some people have relatively shallow curves, while others have very curvaceous spines; each may function well if the curves are in a harmonious balance with one another and with the rest of the body.

When the curves of the spine are balanced in relation to one another, with each curve transitioning smoothly into the next, we call this a *neutral* position. Because this is the optimal position for spinal function, the spine likes to be in this neutral position most of the time. When we sit, stand, walk about, exercise, or sleep, the spine functions best in this neutral position. However, in order to maintain healthy spinal curves, we need to move our backs outside the range of these neutral curves for brief periods of time each day, a task that daily yoga practice will accomplish superbly. When the spine is healthy it doesn't matter if we slouch occasionally, as long as we have the choice to return to a more balanced position. But if we spend our entire lives in positions that compromise the integrity of our spines—bent into our car, hunched over our desk, and collapsed on an overly soft mattress at night— this causes a gradual but nonetheless dramatic degeneration of the spine's structure.

Spinal Integrity

The spinal column can be compared to a string of pearls. In a pearl necklace of value the beads are separated by tiny knots that act as spacers between the precious orbs, preventing them from rubbing and scratching each other. In the human body the spacers between the spinal vertebrae are the spongy intervertebral discs, which absorb shock and separate one bone from another. Each disc has a tough outer layer, much like a woven basket, called the *annulus* and a gel-like center called the *pulposus.* After the second decade of life these fibrocartilaginous discs have no direct blood supply and remain effective cushions only so long as they receive nutrition and moisture from the surrounding tissue.[3] Through a process of squeezing and soaking, the discs absorb nutrients and fluids much as a sponge does when pressed and released. Called *imbibition*, this process prevents the discs from losing resiliency and becoming narrow. Movement stimulates imbibition by compressing and releasing the discs. Moving the spine in all possible planes—forward, back, sideways, and in rotation, is a means of maintaining its flexibility and mobility.

The bones and joints of the spine are both held together and *held apart* by the strong ligaments that connect bone to bone. This fibrous tissue, in combination with the shape and angle of the joint surfaces, determines the specific plane of motion in which each joint can move. Joints require space and lubrication to function correctly, and the ligaments together with the tensile support of the spinal muscles serve to create space between the vertebrae, giving the spine its integrity as a mobile structure.

The space within the spinal column is not only important for movement, it is essential for the life-sustaining action of the central nervous system. As the spinal cord exits the brain, it sweeps through the central canal of the vertebrae, sending vital electrical conducting nerves out from the central branch to innervate the internal organs and the muscles of the body. If the central spinal canal were to become too narrow, as it does in some disease processes, the spinal cord would be impinged. And if the spaces between the vertebrae diminish, the exiting nerves can be painfully pinched, causing a disruption in the communication between the central nervous system and other parts of the body. This is why space is one of the most necessary conditions for health and ease in the spine. When you dangle a pearl necklace having all the beads well spaced, each pearl stays where it should regardless of whether you hang it upside down or curl it into a series of rings for storage in your jewelry box. When you take it out, it still has its original integrity. If we bend backward and do so by crushing the bones together, not only will it hurt while we are doing the movement, the spine may be quite altered when we return to a neutral position. Similarly, if we always compress the discs through poor sitting, standing, and movement habits, we place too much strain on one part of the disc, eventually causing the strong outer coating or annulus of the disc to tear or herniate. When this happens, the gel-like center is pressed out of the disc, which initially can cause severe pain and eventually causes loss of mobility and healthy function in that part of the spine.

In yoga practice the neutral position of the spine acts as a central motif for all other movement. The large majority of the postures ask us to maintain this neutral position, with the neutral spine being the precondition for the more specific actions we wish to do. While the more advanced postures may reverse the curves dramatically for brief periods of time, they are almost always followed by movements that return us to a neutral central axis. The ultimate test of a healthy back is the ability to sit in meditation for long periods of time with complete ease.

Spinal Elongation and Riding the Breath

While the position of our spine is important, simply finding a balanced position is not enough. To bring life to the back we must be able to move force through it. Just as a fountain is an inert object until we run water through it, so, too, the spine lacks vitality until it is brought to life by the combined forces of gravity, the breath, and our directed intention.

The movement of the spine with the breath is essentially the same in all postures. Once you know how to elongate your spine in one position, you can apply this knowledge to every movement that you do. If you lie on your belly and observe your back and breath (or better yet, observe someone else lying prone), you will find that the spine moves like an accordion with your breath (Figures 15 and 16). As you breathe the two ends of the spine alternately condense toward your waist, or center of gravity, and then release in both directions away from your center of gravity. Depending on your relationship to gravity and the position you are in, the elongation phase may take place on either the inhalation or the exhalation. Rather than follow a rule, simply notice which phase of the breath *asks* the spine to elongate or condense and then allow it to happen.

The release and elongation of the spine comes through relaxation rather than effort. While it is possible to reinforce this elongation through directing your intention, you cannot create the release any more than a surfer can create a wave. When you release, it is like opening up the gate to a dam. As you open the gate the current of the breath surges through the spine. All that is left to do is to ride the wave and let the breath move the spine.

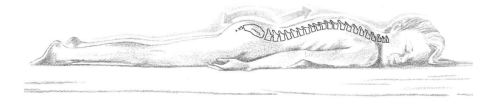

15. *Inhalation*

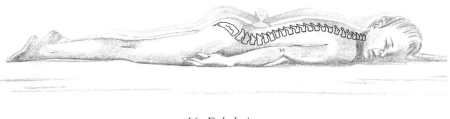

16. *Exhalation*

15 *(Inhalation)* & 16 *(Exhalation)*. *Spinal Elongation: As you breathe in and out, the spine elongates and condenses in unison with your breath. This central mobility will allow you to feel and move from the core of your body, whether you are standing, sitting, or in a yoga posture.*

∽ INQUIRY ∽

Finding Your Neutral Spine

Stand with your feet hips-width apart. Close your eyes and visualize your brain inside the vault of your skull. Imagine the long tail of the brain (your spinal cord) as it exits the brain and sweeps down through the central spinal canal of your back in a series of smooth, sensuous curves. As you scan through your spinal cord, from brain to lower back, imagine the vertebrae of your spinal column like beads around this central thread. Notice if there are any areas where the beads are jammed together or rotated, and if there are any abrupt transitions between the segments of the spine. With the same care you would take if you were moving delicate china, gently adjust the bones around the central thread of the spinal cord until they feel equally spaced. Feel if any of the vertebrae are pressing or abrading the spinal cord, and gently adjust your position until your spine feels light and fine. Take extra care around the base of the skull, where the spinal cord exits the brain, because this is an area where the neck can become chronically compressed. Also pay special attention to your lower back and the transition between your lumbar curve and your sacrum. Create smooth transitions between all the segments of your back. Now explore walking and sitting, maintaining this neutral position of the spine. If you are already familiar with yoga postures, practice an *asana* having the back in a neutral position, and see if you can sustain the clear neutral position of your spine throughout your practice.

∽ INQUIRY ∽

Spinal Elongation and Riding the Breath

Stand with your feet hips-width apart. Begin by balancing your weight over your feet. Then balance the center of your pelvis over the feet. Now center your chest over your pelvis. Last, align the center of your head over your chest. Imagine each central point like a floating planet hovering over the one below it.

Then focus your attention on your exhalation. As you breathe out, feed the weight of your legs and feet into the ground. Feel yourself growing roots down into the ground. As you start to release the spine from the core down toward the earth, the most amazing thing begins to happen. As you exhale, the spine above the waist begins to ascend lightly. When you exhale, both actions occur together—the downward release and the upward ascent. If you cannot feel it, try bending your knees, and experiment with your pelvic, chest, and head positions. The pelvis may be slung under, or the chest may be hanging behind the line of gravity, placing themselves outside the central conduit of the rebounding action. If you are not sure of where your body is in space, place your back against the wall so you can feel your buttocks, upper back, and the back of your skull lightly touching the wall. This will prevent you from coming too far off the vertical axis. Keep your breath moving, and allow the spine to alternately elongate and condense. The coiling action of the condensing phase creates the conditions for the uncoiling action of the elongating phase.

Now try an *asana* that you know, and apply the principles of spinal elongation. You'll find that whether you are sitting, bending forward, or extending into an arc, your spine is alternately pulsing from condensation to elongation. It may take some time to learn how to elongate your spine using gravity as a friend and the breath as the mover. Be patient. Once you have mastered this simple movement you will be able to go to the core of any movement, no matter how seemingly elaborate and complex.

The Principle in Practice

∼ When working with any posture, ask, "Where does my spine need to be to catch the wave of the breath?" Experiment with your position until you feel the breath rolling through the spine.

∼ A tight core prevents spinal elongation. Check that your belly is mobile in every *asana*.

∼ Everyone has areas of the spine that become blocked. These blocked areas prevent elongation. Make a note of your tight spots and spend a little time in each practice session working on movements that open these segments.

5. Support
Foundations of Support: Structural Building Blocks

Whatever touches the ground becomes the foundation of support for each asana.

Whatever part of the body touches the ground becomes the structural base of support. This base dictates what the rest of the body can or cannot do. When support is lacking in the base of a movement, the structures higher up compensate by support*ing* rather than being support*ed*. When the hands, feet, sitting bones, elbows, or head make contact with the ground, it is essential that we distribute the weight of the body evenly through this base. Equal weight distribution at the base creates equal distribution of stress, both in the contacting surface and in the structures supported above the base.

Imagine what it would be like to wear a pair of shoes with the right heel an inch higher than the left. After a short time you would begin to feel strain in one ankle and then in one knee. After a few days one hip would begin to ache, and then one side of your back would start to feel tight and compressed. After a few weeks the shoulder on that side would feel painful and you would find yourself unable to turn your neck evenly. After a month you would have a chronic headache that you could trace back through the zigzag of compensations from the top on down to your mismatched shoes. In chemistry, enzymes can be used to catalyze a series of reactions, with each reaction being activated by the successive products of the previous one, eventually resulting in an amplification of the initial response. In every posture or movement, the way we contact the ground sets off a similar cascade effect.

As a beginning student it can be difficult to know whether you are moving the spine evenly or whether the head is centered because you cannot see these structures. But you usually *can* see and sometimes even touch the supporting base of the pose. When you put your hands on the floor and practice the Downward-Facing Dog, you may not be able to feel whether your weight is centered in your shoulders, but you can see and feel whether your weight is centered in your hands. Thus not only can you use the base of the pose to balance the rest of the body, but you can read what the rest of the body is doing from the action of the base support. If, for instance, the weight always tends to fall on the outside of the wrist, this alerts you that you tend to use the outer muscles of the shoulder more than the inner ones. If you tend to collapse the arches of your feet, this tells you something about the inner rotation of your knees and the collapse through your lower back.

Although we'll go into bases of support in more detail in each *asana* section, for now consider that the action of your hands will affect your arms and shoulders; the action of your feet will affect your knees, hips, and trunk; and the action of your pelvis will most directly affect your spinal column. Parts of the body above the base of support will mirror the action of their supporting structures.

～ INQUIRY ～

The Cascade Effect of the Foundation

This is just one simple exercise to demonstrate the radical cascade effect that occurs from the foundation of the *asana* all the way through the body. Stand with your feet hips-width apart. Begin by rocking your weight onto your heels and remaining there. Stay for a minute or longer and feel the effects of this stance in your ankles, knees, hips, and back. Notice whether the muscles on the front and back of the body are working equally or whether one side of the body is more dominant. Now rock onto your toes and remain with your weight forward. Stay for a minute or more and notice the difference in the way your ankles, knees, and hips feel. Continue scanning up your body. Then experiment with rocking onto the outsides of your feet, followed by standing on the inside edges of your feet. Then center your weight over your feet so that it is balanced equally over the entire surface of the foot. Compare these sensations with the ones you felt when your weight was behind, in front, or to the side of this central balance.

The Principle in Practice
- ∼ Whenever you are having difficulty in a posture, check and adjust the base of the pose first.
- ∼ The broader the base of support, the more stable you will be.
- ∼ Tension in the upper body indicates a lack of support in the lower body.

6. Align
Lines of Force: Alignment and Sequential Flow

Alignment is the clear sequential flow of force through the body.

A dry riverbed winds its way through a deep valley. Without water, the river has little effect upon the gravel bed or the rocks and boulders in its path. When the river flows with water, then and only then does it have power to change and to carry things from one place to another. The river can now move rocks, wear away at boulders, and even change its very course, cutting into and altering the surrounding banks. In the same way, *asanas* do not transform the body until we can effectively move force through them. When we align ourselves in a yoga *asana* we find a harmonious relationship between the parts of the body so that force can be conducted into, through, and beyond the body into space. As force sequences through the body it opens the spaces between joints, elongates muscles, and clears a pathway for energy to flow freely.

Alignment is not, as is commonly thought, a static position that we hold. Nor is alignment limited to straight and linear relationships. Rather, aligning the body is an art composed of two steps. The first step in aligning ourselves is to find a cooperative relationship between the parts of the body. This can be as simple as rotating the foot in the same direction as the knee. When we find this cooperative relationship, the parts of the body are in agreement with one another about the action to be performed. The foot agrees with the knee and therefore they can now move in unified action. The arrangement of the structure determines where force can and cannot flow, just as the course of a riverbed determines the flow of the water through it.

The second step in aligning ourselves is much more dynamic, and like most simple things it can be the hardest to understand. Now that we have positioned ourselves, the body is ready to be animated by first allowing natural force to move through it. You have already done this in the previous inquiries on yielding and elongation. Here we take the work a step further, so that we are actively engaged in *directing* force through the body to reinforce the natural openings that are already there, and to connect our movement with the environment: the earth below, the space around us, and the sky above. I call this second step *engaged alignment* to distinguish it from the mere act of mechanical placement.

The first stage of alignment is like laying down a railway track, aligning each segment of the track with the next so the train can run in a smooth path. The second step of engaging the alignment involves running force through the body. By following the natural line of the bones and respecting the direction in which each joint moves, we find that alignment is intrinsic to our very structure. If the muscles hang off the bones and the joints lack integrity, the bones become like railway tracks that are misaligned. When the train (force) travels along the tracks, it moves side to side or off the track rather than in a clear, efficient motion. When you yield your weight into a supporting surface, the bones take the supporting role and act as clear conducting rods. As force flows along the bones and across the joint spaces positioned through your conscious directional intent, the muscles begin to follow suit, streaming parallel to the bones like the current of wind that follows after a train has run down the tracks.

We *engage* our alignment in two main ways. We can yield and push against a supporting surface with a peripheral limb (hands, feet, head, sitting bones) and direct the rebounding force through our center and out through the opposite periphery. Or we can initiate a movement by reaching through one of our limbs into space and following through with the rest of the body. When a baseball player reaches to catch a ball, the rest of his body follows his intent. In a Headstand we yield and push with the head and elbows against the ground and direct the rebounding force up through the body, completing the movement by reaching up into space with the feet. In all movements *yield underlies push and push underlies reach*. Usually if we push from one end of our structure, we must reach with the opposite end to complete the movement. As you sit in your chair you must yield and push downward with your sitting bones to create a rebound through your spine. This rebound can be further supported by an active reach upward through the head (Figure 17).

Fortunately, it is easy to test good alignment. All we need do is challenge the alignment by exerting an external force through the structure. If there are poor relationships between structures, as you exert force through the body you will see and feel a "break" or wobble in the areas that are badly aligned. Experiment with the following inquiry to find your alignment in this simple *asana*.

17. *Engaged Alignment*

∼ INQUIRY ∼

Following the Line of the Bones

Place your hands shoulders-width apart and at shoulder height on a wall. Spread your fingers wide and slowly begin to walk your feet away from the wall until your back forms a tabletop position and your feet are directly under your hips.

Yield the surface of your hands against the wall and then begin to push the wall away. As you push back, feel the force moving through your arms, straightening the elbows and moving into the shoulders. Take a breath in and, as you breathe out, allow the force to travel into your spine and torso. Reinforce this natural elongation by continuing to push back through the wall and actively reaching through your sitting bones and tail.

Experiment with the angle of your arms and torso to find the clearest line of force through the body. Because everyone's body proportions are unique, your best alignment will be different from another person's. To feel the difference between the first and second stages of alignment, notice what happens when you simply assume the position of the tabletop without sending force through your body. This inquiry should clarify the difference between finding an aligned position and engaging the alignment by moving force through the body.

In Figure 18 the model in Half-Dog Pose is in a well-aligned position. Notice how her arms form a clear line from the palms to the shoulders and her torso follows this line. She is actively pushing into the wall and reaching back through her tail and sitting bones, creating space between all the bones on each outgoing breath. If a helper sends force through her sitting bones by pressing into the pelvis, he feels a clear, uninterrupted line from sitting bones to hands. Even if the helper presses very strongly, there are no breaks or wobbles anywhere in the body. The strength of her position is created not by sheer muscular energy but by the sound functional relationship among all the parts of her body.

In Figure 19 the model is hyperextending in all her joints. Notice that she sags at the elbows, and that there is a zigzag line between her arms and her torso. If we press into this structure, we will feel a "jiggle" where the breaks in the alignment occur—at the wrist, elbow, shoulder, and in the spine. If we increase our pressure, the model will be unable to sustain the position, not because her individual muscles are weak, but because her muscles and bones are in a poor relationship with one another and cannot function effectively.

In Figure 20 the model is unable to bend from the hips because of the stiffness in her legs and spine. Notice that the back rises above the line of the arms and is outside the conduit of force. If we press through this structure we will feel a "jiggle" in the parts of the back that are not able to follow the line of the arms. This person could improve her alignment by raising her arms higher on the wall so that the angle of the arms more clearly matches the flexibility of the spine and hips (Figure 21). Although this is a more elementary position, her

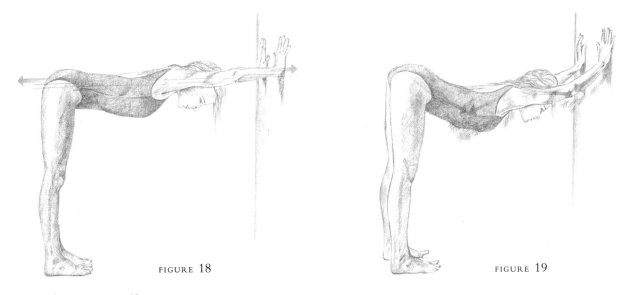

FIGURE 18   FIGURE 19

18–21. *Alignment in Half-Dog*

force can now run clearly from her arms through her spine, and therefore she is better aligned.

The Principle in Practice

～ Pain is a warning signal that you are poorly aligned. Pain and good alignment are mutually exclusive conditions.

～ Modify your alignment in every pose to reflect your present flexibility and skill level rather than forcing your body to conform to an ideal position. Your body is unique and what you need to do to be well aligned will differ from another person.

～ Good alignment allows you to do more with less effort. Poor alignment requires more energy to sustain.

7. Engage
Engage the Whole Body: The Democratic Body Community

Every body system has its own unique function, expression, and associated quality of consciousness and is interdependent with every other system in the body. In embodied spiritual practice we nurture democracy within the body community as a way of creating balance, harmony, and freedom (Figures 22–27).

The ancient yogis had a profound awareness of the human system based on their personal experiential mapping of the body-mind entity. Their geographical mappings of the body territory identified subtle layers and energetic forces that objective Western science does not as yet recognize. When we visit a country, we are

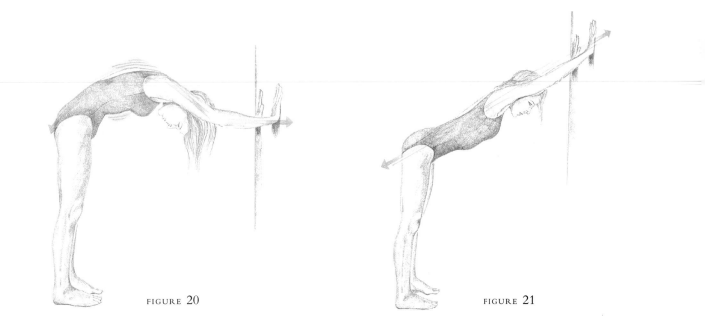

FIGURE 20   FIGURE 21

affected by the local, state, and national laws of that particular culture. Just because we cannot "see" these laws does not mean they do not exist. In the same way, the body is organized and coordinated by forces we may not be able to reduce into tangible objects but that nonetheless have a powerful and pervading influence over everything we do.

Much of the written information about yoga that has been passed down to us from India is of an esoteric nature, giving us few practical clues as to how to access these subtle systems for ourselves. To this day, many practices are transmitted only through the oral tradition of teacher to a carefully selected student, and thus much of the most vital information has been lost or forgotten. As new paradigms for health and spirituality have emerged in the West, we are discovering our own means of locating, defining, and directly experiencing profound aspects of the body-mind entity. This is a hopeful sign that we may be able to recover much of this lost knowledge.

The following sections of this book owe much to the inspiring work of Bonnie Bainbridge Cohen, director of the School for Body-Mind Centering in Amherst, Massachusetts.[4] As a seminal researcher of experiential anatomy and human developmental movement patterns, Bainbridge Cohen has researched the theoretical and experiential ways in which the different body systems contribute to the quality of our movement and consciousness. Her writings, and the influence of this method, have given me a more tangible language to describe many of the systems that until now have been hidden within the esoteric yoga tradition.

Our bodies are made up of systems, each of which has its own function, expressive quality, and associated consciousness. In the West our primary focus has been on those structures and systems that we can see, so our awareness of the body has remained largely superficial. The musculoskeletal system, the organ system, the endocrine and nervous system, the fluid system, and other systems such as the fas-

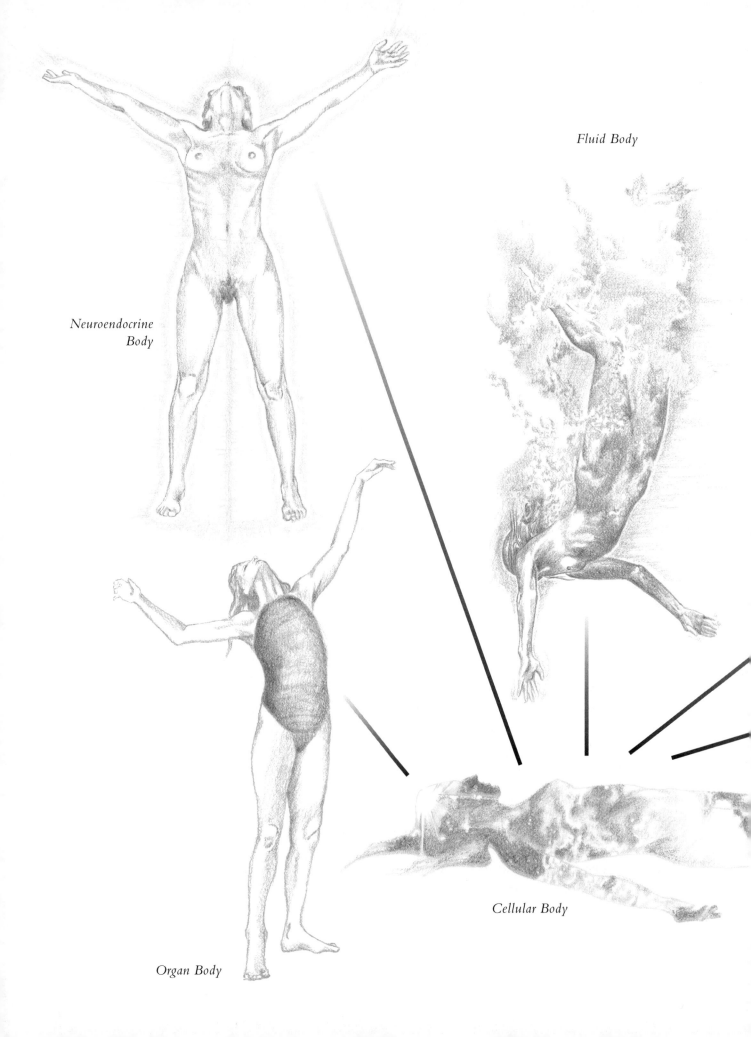

Neuroendocrine Body

Fluid Body

Organ Body

Cellular Body

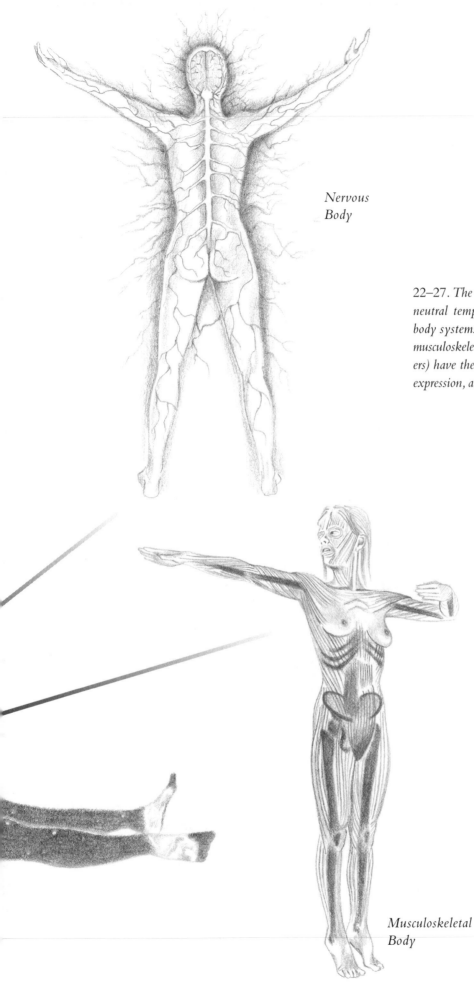

*Nervous
Body*

22–27. *The Whole Body Community: From the neutral template of the cellular body the other body systems arise. The fluid, organ, glandular, musculoskeletal, and nervous systems (among others) have their own structure, function, quality of expression, and consciousness.*

*Musculoskeletal
Body*

cial connective tissue, fat, and the skin comprise the major members of the body community. Each of us has individual preferences and proclivities to live in some systems more than others. Some people tend to be very "highly strung," indicating a tendency to draw heavily upon the nervous system. Others tend to be very easy-going, quick to adapt, and smooth in their movements, revealing a natural ability to draw support from the fluid systems. There is nothing wrong with these constitutional tendencies, but they can limit our choices and our ability to respond effectively to new situations. When we become aware of, and begin to live from, unfamiliar aspects of ourselves we find that our range of expression expands, as do our choices.

A complete study of all the body systems is beyond the scope of this book. There are, however, a number of systems that are of particular relevance to the yoga practitioner. These are the cellular, musculoskeletal, fluid, organ, and neuro-endocrine systems. Although balancing the nervous system is central to yoga practice, I have chosen to offer access to this system through the other systems. The Western model for learning about these systems has been entirely theoretical and based upon cognitive understanding—one studies biology, anatomy, physiology as if studying an external object. In yoga practice we attempt to visualize, sense, and *feel* the actuality of these systems—we not only become familiar with the map, we also take a walk through the territory over and over again until we know it like the back of our hand. This ongoing experiential practice broadens the spectrum of our consciousness from a limited outline to a comprehensive three-dimensional picture of who we are. At first this may seem far-fetched, but even the casual runner stretching after a morning jog notices that after a few days of stretching and sensing the state of her hamstring muscles she becomes familiar with their tone, tissue quality, and function and can easily detect when the fiber has been pulled or damaged in some way. In yoga we take this practice much deeper, sensing, feeling, and moving from more subtle dimensions of the body such as the internal organs, the glands, or the circulation of fluids. We begin to read the action of the body and mind, developing a fluent "body literacy."

While these body systems are organized through a Western paradigm, they give us a foothold into the more subtle dimensions of the body described in Eastern traditions. The major difference between this process and mere objectification so common to our culture is that we work with *felt* somatic experience. The difference between these two methods is like the difference between studying a foreign country from a book and living within that country. The pictures in the guidebook, the language texts, and the maps of famous city streets rarely give us any true idea of the nature of the place we are studying. It is not until we are actually there, tasting the food, feeling the climate, learning the customs, hearing the language, and following the rhythm of daily life that the essential nature of the place is revealed. In the same way, knowing the names of all the muscles, organs, and nerves in the body does not give us any real sense of their essential nature. We have to live *in* the body to know it.

The following inquiries take you on a guided tour of some of the body systems. As you become more intimate with the felt experience of these systems, explore how they can offer their support within your yoga practice.

The Cellular System

Key Attributes: being, matrix, simplicity, neutrality, pure potential, rest

Structure and Qualities: Every cell has a basic structure. The cell has an outer semipermeable membrane that encloses the jellylike fluid cytoplasm, which is 70 to 80 percent water. Inside the cell are specialized structures that carry on the work of protein synthesis, the generation of energy, and cell division. At the center of each cell is the nucleus that carries the genetic material which determines your unique characteristics. As the human embryo develops, cells differentiate to take on specialized tasks and roles. Some become nerve cells, others bone and connective-tissue cells, while others become muscle cells. The structure and arrangement of these cells determines their function within your body.

There are billions of cells in the human body, and every cell in your body breathes, taking in oxygen and giving out carbon dioxide and by-products. It is the cells that desire the breath, and ultimately this is the force that drives the breathing process. Cells need energy, and they acquire this energy through the nutrients we eat and through a constant supply of oxygen. When air enters our bodies, it takes a circuitous path through the body, from the lungs into the blood, from large blood vessels to small blood vessels, until the oxygen carried on the back of hemoglobin in the blood reaches the tiny thin-walled capillaries surrounding the cells. Oxygen and nutrients are delivered to the cells, and the cells give carbon dioxide and by-products back into the blood capillaries. This bluish deoxygenated blood flows back though the veins, traveling into larger and larger blood vessels until it reaches the heart, where it is once again pumped out to the lungs to receive new oxygen.

Every cell in the body alternately expands and condenses in an ongoing rhythmic state of respiration. When we are aware of our bodies at this most basic level of organization, we are physically locating the mind in the ground of our being. The cells are the ground matrix from which all other states, both physical and psychological, evolve. The cellular level of awareness is the field from which all other intentions form.[5] Cells represent the undifferentiated state of form and being. When we bring our awareness into the cells, we enter an unbounded state of consciousness that is free from ideas of separate identity, differences, and categorization. Whenever we wish to return to our sense of self, we must enter this physiological substratum. As we become more skilled, we are able to sustain an ongoing connection with our matrix. This connection with the matrix is the physical organization of meditation and self-reflection, an essential base in all yoga practices. To experience the cells, then, we must allow the habitual background noise of the mind and the distraction of activity to diminish so that the quieter voice of the cells can be heard. This is the process of meditation.

～ INQUIRY ～

The Cellular Body

Lie facedown on a soft surface with your head turned to one side. If this is not comfortable for your neck, place a few pillows or folded blankets under your torso so that your chest is slightly higher than your head. Take a few moments to settle into a comfortable position, allowing your weight to be received by the earth (see Figure 230, page 239).

Begin to sense into your breathing, following the path of your breath into your lungs. Let your mind travel on the back of the breath, moving deep into the lungs, deeper and deeper until you find yourself in the tiny alveoli air sacs. Then comes a miraculous moment. The oxygen that is in your breath is transferred from these bubblelike sacs into your blood. In an instant the breath is changed from a gas to a fluid medium. Follow the movement of your fluid breath from the capillaries into the heart. Feel the strong pumping action of the heart as it propels the blood into the body, causing the blood to travel into the furthermost regions of the body. As you follow the blood, eventually it trickles into tiny capillaries so small that the blood cells must squeeze to move through. Here the blood gives up its precious cargo to the cells.

Enter your cells. Expanding, condensing, and resting in an ongoing shimmering rhythm. Sense and feel yourself as this vital whole matrix. What is your personal experience of your cellular body? What is your mind-body state when you become more present to this level of your organization? Allow yourself to descend into the quiet stillness and pure state of potential. Rest, recuperate, and enjoy simply being. When you are ready to sit up, bring this pervasive presence with you into all your actions.

The System in Practice

～ The pause between two breaths is an entryway into the cellular level of yourself. As you fill the pause with your awareness, the pause becomes more spacious. Relax into the silence of the pause.

～ Imagine yourself as the sky, and all the fleeting sensations and feelings that pass through you as drifting clouds. Allow the sensations to arise, but sustain your awareness of yourself as the omnipresent sky.

～ When you become confused or hurried, take a minute to sit still and be with your breath. As you breathe, count down from ten to one on each exhalation. Imagine yourself returning back to your center as you do so.

The Musculoskeletal System

Key Attributes: support and power, directed action, specificity and clarity, manifested intention

Structure and Qualities: As we evolved from life in the primordial sea to life on land, our bodies had to adapt to the new challenges of moving on solid ground and the special forces of gravity. This evolution from amorphous, "boneless" fluidity to the crystallization of form we call our skeleton, today, provides us with a central internal architecture that, together with the containing skin sheath and all the other body systems, allows us to carry our own oceanic system wherever we go (Figure 28).

The bones are our most enduring body substance, surviving as evidence of our lives long after the rest of the physical body has disintegrated. When alive, the bones are a pinkish white on the outside and deep red within.[6] Elastic collagen fibrils give bone its plasticity and resilience while densely packed calcium, phosphorus, and other trace minerals give it its solidity and strength. Bones grow in response to bearing weight and the movements we perform. Like the skin, they continually replace themselves throughout adult life, remodeling taking place at different rates in different areas. Some parts of the thigh bone are replaced almost every four months[7] while other parts of the skeleton are not entirely replaced over a lifetime. Inactivity can damage bones as much as stress—a broken leg in a cast can lose up to 30 percent of its calcium content during a few weeks of bed rest.[8]

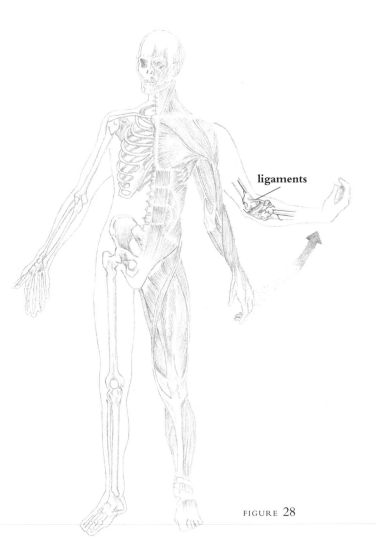

ligaments

The bones of the skeleton articulate at joints, some deep and stable like the hip, others shallow and unstable like the shoulder. The joints are held together by fibrous ligamental tissue that serves to define the range and direction of movement. This alone would not be enough to make the skeleton a stable structure, as anyone who has ever handled an anatomical model will know. It is not until we complete the picture with the six hundred muscles attached to the bones by means of strong tendons that the skeleton gains its integrity and can now be animated through the action of the nervous system into an astonishing repertoire of movements, ranging from the gross action of walking to the subtle nuance of a facial expression.

The musculoskeletal system acts as our most primary and tangible body mover. Because of its extraordinary virtuosity and the tangible nature

FIGURE 28

of its existence, the musculoskeletal system tends to dominate our perception and experience of the body, which in modern times has reached extreme levels of obsession. For many people the practice of hatha yoga is exclusively associated with increasing the flexibility of the musculoskeletal system, progress being measured through the mastery of ever more difficult postures. While this simplification allowed yoga to get a foothold in the West, the mechanization of hatha yoga into a sophisticated form of calisthenics has, at times, drowned out the voices of other members of the body community and masked the primary purpose of the practice.

In a democratic body community the strong action of the muscles and bones is balanced and modulated by the other members of the body community. As you will see in the inquiries to come, the fluids, organs, and glands offer substantial support for movement as well as giving you a greater range of expression than would be possible when only one body system is allowed to dominate.

～ INQUIRY ～

The Mover and the Moved

It's important to have the support of your musculoskeletal system, but too much effort and muscular tension can prevent the free movement of the breath and fluids through the body. To find out how to calibrate the degree of muscular activity, try this inquiry.

Stand or sit, and extend your arms out to your sides with your hands in line with your shoulders. Note how much effort you need to exert to create lightness in the extension of your arms but still feel the breath gently oscillating them. The oscillation will cause the arms to alternately release back toward your center and then away from your center. The arms may also move slightly up and down as well as rotate in and out. Look down the length of one arm and see the movements the breath is making through your arm. Now intensify the degree of muscular effort, using far more than you need to extend the arms. Grip the muscles tightly to the bones. At what point do you feel the oscillation of the breath cease moving freely through your arms? Let your arms hang limp, and notice if they are effective carriers for the breath's movement. Experiment until you find the optimal balance between effort and release, where your arms are extended but still moving in response to your breath.

Now try this inquiry in a yoga *asana* that you know well. Notice how the degree of effort varies from moment to moment and how different areas of your body need to be more supportive than others, depending on the movement you attempt. Whenever you can no longer feel the oscillation of the breath, you know you are outside the optimum threshold of muscular tension. This is true for all postures and movements.

The System in Practice

～ In the first few breaths of entering a yoga *asana* notice where your mind goes. The mind is usually drawn to areas of excess tension. Exhale and relax from the center of that place. Release.

～ Notice *where* you tire first while practicing a yoga *asana*. This may be an indication that you overuse or incorrectly use that muscle, that you are weak in that area, or that that particular part of the body is not functionally integrated with the rest of the body.

～ In every *asana* ask where you need support and where you need to release. As a general rule whatever part of the body is in contact with the ground usually supports, while those parts exposed to space generally release.

The Fluid System

Key Attributes: flow, circulation, transformation, smooth transitions, ease, lubrication, buoyancy, and fun

Structure and Qualities: Our fluids have a composition very similar to ocean water. So it is not a far leap to say our human body is an encapsulation of the primordial sea from which we came. All the fluids in the body have one oceanic source—the interstitial fluid. Composed of a matrix of collagen fiber bundles, tiny proteoglycan filaments, and water, the interstitium is a gel-like medium that suspends and surrounds the cells, giving tissue its firm tensional strength. Although of a gel consistency, the interstitial fluid has the remarkable ability to transport substances almost as quickly as water itself. As fluid gushes, pulses, streams, and trickles throughout the body, transporting nutrients and oxygen, it crosses thin membranes, and in doing so it changes into blood, lymph, cellular fluid, cerebrospinal fluid, or synovial fluid. When we are born, our bodies are composed of up to 70 percent fluid. By maintaining free circulation of fluid in the body, we can stay youthful and juicy as we age.

As we think of ourselves, so we become. The awkward child labeled "clumsy" begins to think of himself as clumsy and fulfills the label with each glass of milk he spills. So, too, if we think of ourselves as solid and unchangeable, as statues of fired clay rather than the moist, pliable medium that we are, we find ourselves hardening into a fixed identity. Consider that imagining yourself as a body of water is not pure fancy, it is the truth of your physical existence (Figure 29). You *are* fluid.

Each fluid in the body has its own function, expressive quality, and consciousness—from the vibrant earthiness of the staccato pulse of the arterial blood, to the sustained ethereal flow of the cerebrospinal fluid that surrounds and lubricates the brain and spinal cord; from the slippery jiggle of the synovial fluid of the joints, to the periorgan fluid that surrounds the organs, to the calm serenity of the fluid pooled inside the home of our cells. While it is of great value to explore each in detail, we will limit ourselves to a generalized awareness of the fluids as a whole.

When we see someone who moves with grace and smooth seamless transitions,

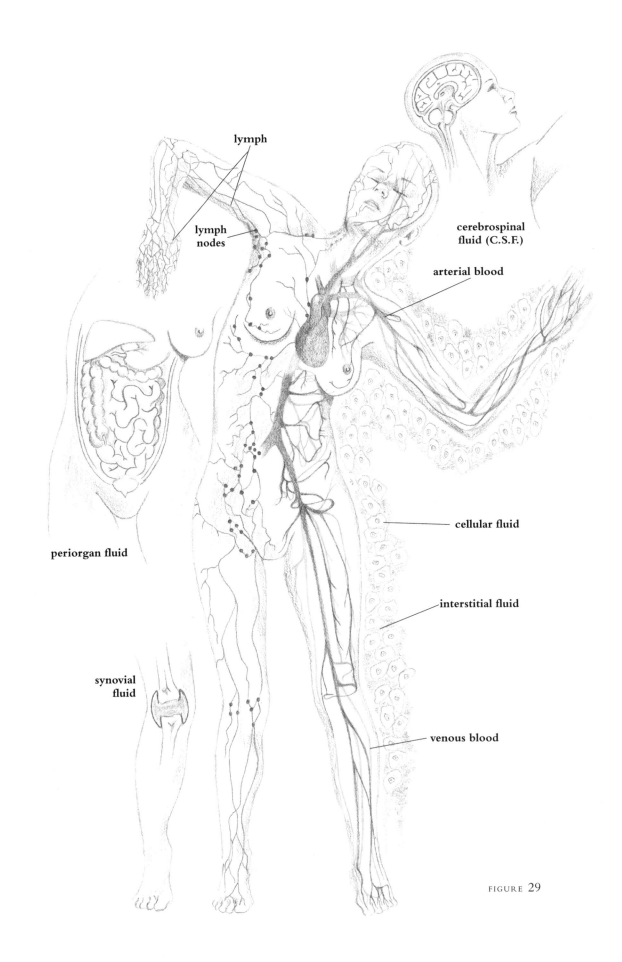

lymph

lymph
nodes

cerebrospinal
fluid (C.S.F.)

arterial blood

cellular fluid

interstitial fluid

periorgan fluid

synovial
fluid

venous blood

FIGURE 29

we are seeing the support of the fluids in action. A fluid person's actions seem to flow, undulate, and glide, each movement connected to the next. One of the main properties of water is its ability to provide cohesion for other elements. Dry, dusty earth falls through our hands, but when mixed with water it has pliable form that we can shape. When we do not live in the watery element of ourselves, our movement becomes dry and brittle, disconnected and segmented. The growing lack of fluidity so common in older people today is not a foregone conclusion of aging. It is true that we do lose some fluid content as we age, but the premature stiffness and immobility seen in modern people as young as thirty is more the result of living without the conscious presence of fluidic support, which can be compared to dying of thirst while sitting in the middle of an oasis.

The ability to adapt and change is a quality of fluid embodiment. Just as water conforms to the shape of the container it is placed in, the person with a fluid nature is able to adjust to new and oftentimes unexpected and unfamiliar situations with ease. Certain cultures are more or less fluidic in nature. When traveling in Central America, I have been impressed by the accommodating nature of the people and their ability to accept and even welcome the unexpected. In contrast, Americans and European peoples tend to expect life to be a certain way, and when inevitably met with delays and changes of plan, they tend to respond by fixing, defining, and defending their version of reality, even if this version does little to create ease within themselves or the people around them. Just as fluid lubricates a hinge, when we live and move fluidly, we are able to open to change with less resistance and difficulty.

～ INQUIRY ～

The Fluidic Body

Lie facedown on a soft surface. If this is uncomfortable for your neck or back, place a few soft pillows or folded blankets underneath your torso so that your chest and belly are slightly elevated above your head and limbs (see Figure 230, page 239). Let a few deep exhalations out through your mouth, allowing your weight to settle into the ground. Let everyday concerns drop away. When your breathing becomes quiet and still, you are ready to begin.

Close your eyes. Imagine yourself as a body of water encapsulated by your skin. Feel the buoyant softness of this internal fluid body. Allow your sense of definition and form to drop away as your hard bony skeleton dissolves into the background of your awareness. Allow to fall away any sense of restriction, tightness, or fixity, and any ideas you have about yourself. As you descend into your internal waters, feel the pulsation of breath moving you. Feel how impulses travel from your core in ripples and how your limbs can become fluid projections from the live center. As you feel an impulse to move, let yourself slither, roll, quiver, and glide. Allow yourself to change level, to roll onto your side or back. Feel the slippery, lubricating support of your fluids, and as you move, allow your body to flow over the ground just as water flows and takes the shape of its container.

Once you have a felt sense of your fluid body, begin to let your skeleton crystallize once again into a pliable internal architecture. Now as you move, feel how this internal form gives your movement direction and specificity, but instead of becoming dry and mechanical in your movements, let your bones be suspended and buoyant within your fluids. As you feel an impulse to move, let the fluid and the skeletal bodies move in intimate concert, feeling how the fluids give your movement ease and fullness. When you are ready, come to a place of stillness and rest. To complete the inquiry, roll over on your side, and as you sit up bring your fluid body with you.

Now explore this balance while you practice a yoga *asana*. Allow the internal scaffolding of your skeleton to be suspended within your fluid body. This will allow you continually to make the tiny shifts and adjustments necessary to find an even stronger alignment. Find a balance between standing strong and remaining open to possibility.

The System in Practice

∼ Shake, jiggle, and roll your body to stimulate the production of synovial fluid in your joints. Do this before and in between movements to loosen and release stiffness.

∼ Focus on smooth transitions while you move from position to position, as a way of sustaining the circulation of fluids.

∼ Select music that makes you feel graceful and flowing. Start your practice with the support of the music and graduate into silence as your practice progresses.

The Organ System

Key Attributes: weight, substance, volume, processing; feelings of slowness, fullness, groundedness, expressiveness, regularity

Structure and Quality: The organs make up the inner contents of your body. By sensitizing yourself to the location, function, sensation, and experience of your internal organs, you can stimulate their healthy working, catch early warning signals of disease, and activate their support for ease in movement and expression (Figures 30 and 31). The organs, some of which are also muscles, like the stomach, are normally considered beyond our conscious control; their function is largely regulated by the parasympathetic branch of the central nervous system. However, the original yogis believed that every part of the human organism had the potential to become conscious, and this is evidenced by our records of some of their remarkable feats, as well as modern biofeedback studies.

When you bring your attention into the core of the body and begin to activate the central support of the organs, this stimulates the parasympathetic part of your nervous system; the part of the nervous system that slows things down and supports

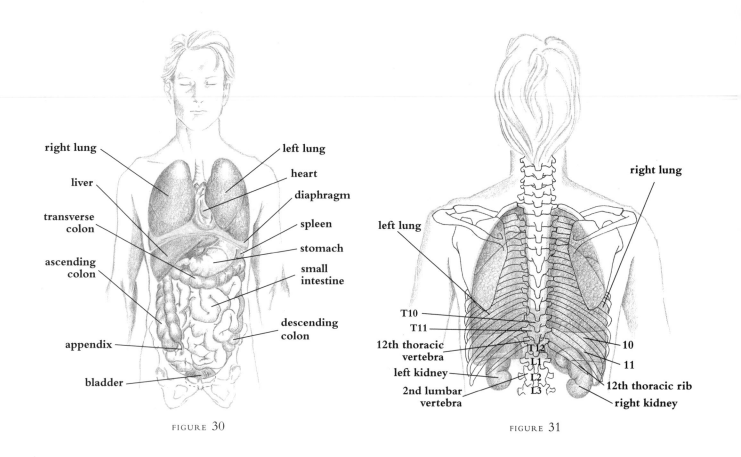

FIGURE 30	FIGURE 31

the processes of digestion, assimilation, and elimination. My own research with yoga students throughout the world has shown that when people become conscious of their inner bodies, their breathing immediately relaxes and deepens and their movement automatically becomes slow and measured. This phenomenon, I believe, is a sign that the parasympathetic aspect of the nervous system is balancing the action of the sympathetic nervous system (the part of the nervous system responsible for the fright, fight, flight, or fake-it response).

When we initiate movement from the core, our inner experience becomes more and more congruent with our outer actions. Postures unfold as a result of an inner opening and expansion that is communicated to the outer container. Rather than being tyrannized by the externally referenced ideas of how far we think we should be able to go or what we should look like in a posture, we begin to listen to the voice of our inner perceptions and trust ourselves to act from them.

Some teachers refer to this sensibility as "moving from the inner body," "moving from the core," or "moving from the center." When we talk about the body in these terms, we are talking about both a definite physical location (the organ system), and a psychological space within ourselves that has no specific locus.

In our yoga practice we can dramatically increase the benefits of the *asanas* by focusing our awareness on these crucial centers of health. While musculoskeletal initiation, support, and alignment are important, the muscles and bones must work in concert with the inner organ system. When we continually overuse and rely on the musculoskeletal system without the underlying cooperation of the organs, we can exhaust ourselves, and we also can injure ourselves through leveraging too strongly from the outside against an unmoving center. In order to sense this more subtle system it is helpful in the beginning to "turn down the volume" of musculoskeletal action. As we let the quieter voice of the inner body be heard, we may find dormant aspects of our consciousness emerging, while the musculoskeletal system has the opportunity for much-needed rest and recuperation.

Every *asana* is an interplay between the inner contents and the outer container of the body, each communicating with and influencing the condition of the other. The challenge of integrating these two systems also shows up in our everyday lives. By focusing on and perceiving the state of the inner body, we can begin to map how sensations correspond to feelings As we become more "internally literate," we can know with certainty what we feel at any given moment and can navigate our actions in the world accordingly. Moving from our deeper selves with this clarity can powerfully impact our personal lives, the lives of those around us, and, ultimately, our surrounding environment.

～ INQUIRY ～

"Organ-ized" Standing/Organ Support

Stand in a relaxed position with your feet hips-width apart. Take a moment to feel the habitual organ-ization of your standing posture. Notice which internal organs seem to collapse or deflate, rotate or torque, and where in your internal structure you feel buoyant, inflated, and centered. Notice that your internal organization influences the arrangement of your frame, and how the set of your bones influences the position of your internal organs.

Now direct your attention into your chest. Notice if your heart and lungs feel expansive or whether they hide inside the cavity of your chest and rib cage. Begin consciously to expand and dilate your heart and lungs by breathing into them, allowing this open posture to emerge gradually from your inner body. As you feel this inner body support, extend your arms up and out to the sides so they are in line with your shoulders. Notice the ease or difficulty that you feel in your arm muscles in this extended position. Now, without changing the position of your arms, let your heart and lungs collapse downward in your chest. Count the seconds it takes before your arm muscles begin to tire. If you are like most people, the arm muscles become fatigued almost immediately without the central support of the heart and lungs. Expand and open

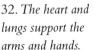
32. *The heart and lungs support the arms and hands.*

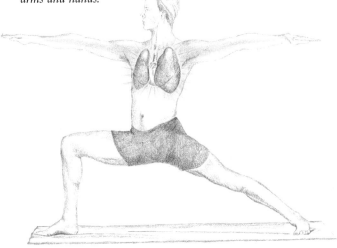

FIGURE 32

your heart and lungs again and notice the support this offers your arms (Figure 32). Do you still believe that your muscles are the central support for your arms?

∼ INQUIRY ∼

The Organ Body Scan

You can do this inquiry as you sit in your chair. Read a paragraph and then take the time to sense and feel. Or you can lie on a soft surface in any position that is comfortable for you and have a friend read the inquiry for you. You may want to divide the inquiry into sections, focusing on one area and using that as a theme for your yoga practice that day. Begin to scan your body, starting with the outermost surface, your skin, and gradually moving through your surface fat, through to your muscles, bones, and inward into the soft center where your organs live.

The Brain and Spinal Cord

Bring your awareness to your head, first sensing and feeling the bony vault of your skull. Inside the cranium lies the soft brain. Go there. Breathe into, around, and from your brain, using your breath fingers to become more intimate with this organ. Feel the state of the brain—does it feel hot, cold, or warm? Does it feel wet, dry, or moist? Does it feel dense or expansive? As you begin to get a better sense of your brain, begin to initiate the turn of your head from the brain itself. Go slowly, letting the weight and volume of the brain slowly loll the head from side to side.

Now let your awareness travel down the tail of the brain into your spinal cord. Follow the tail as it exits the brain at the base of the skull, sweeping down through the narrow spinal canal through your spinal vertebrae. Like a slippery thread winding its way through the central hole of the vertebral beads, the spinal cord moves through the inward curve of your neck, the outward curve of your thoracic or middle spine, and into the arch of your lumbar or lower back, exiting as a brushlike tail of nerves called the *cauda equinine,* or the horse's tail, at about the level of your waist.

Follow the length of the spinal cord, feeling for any places where the beadlike vertebrae press, pinch, or twist upon the central thread of the spine. Notice any areas that feel abraded or places where the cord arches or turns suddenly and notice places where the spinal cord feels smooth and cool and where the transitions from one segment of the spine to the next are smooth.

The Digestive Tract

Now take your awareness into your mouth, the entrance of your digestive system. Take a deep swallow, following the swallow down into your esophagus, ending in your stomach, the place where you break down raw material and ideas. Sense and

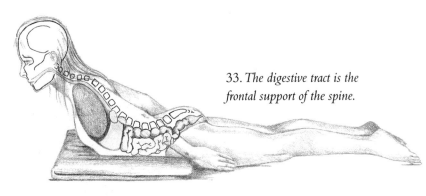

33. *The digestive tract is the frontal support of the spine.*

FIGURE 33

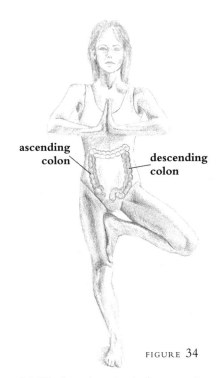

ascending colon

descending colon

FIGURE 34

34. *The large intestine is the energetic support for the legs.*

feel the quality of your stomach, which is both an organ and a muscle. As you breathe into, around, through, and from your stomach, notice if it feels hot, cold or warm, moist or dry. Does it feel full or empty, active and satisfied, or bloated and stagnant? Each time you enter an internal organ, explore by initiating your movement from that organ.

Continue on down through the stomach, entering your small intestine, the winding, slippery tube that makes up the greater portion of your central abdomen. Place your hands there and feel the quality of this internal organ. Does it feel lubricated and smooth, or dry and bloated? Does it feel cold, hot, or warm? Are there any areas that feel congested? Let your breath expand into your abdomen, and notice that as you do so the small intestine slides and rolls, churns and undulates inside the belly.

Now direct your attention to the lower right quadrant of your abdomen. Here the small intestine joins the large intestine via the ileocecal valve. The large intestine encircles the abdomen, traveling up the right side of the abdomen as the ascending colon, across the top of the abdomen as the transverse colon, down the left side as the descending colon, and ending in the sigmoid colon, rectum, and anus. Thus your digestive tract is one long tube from mouth to anus that lies parallel to your spine. It is lined with moist inner "skin" that registers everything you take inside your body. Breathe, feel, and initiate movement from your belly center (Figures 33 and 34).

Heart and Lungs

Now bring your hands onto your chest, feeling for your heartbeat on the left side of your chest. Breathe into your heart, sensing the front, back, and sides of this vital powerhouse. Notice whether the heart feels tight and congested or open and expansive. Does it feel moist or dry, cool or inflamed? As you connect with your heart, also start to sense the state of your lungs, lying on either side of the heart. Breathe into your lungs, noticing if they feel buoyant or heavy, wet or dry. Experiment with changing your chest position, adjusting from the internal structures of your heart and lungs.

Liver, Spleen, and Kidneys

Continue your organ scan, using the illustrations (Figures 30 and 31, page 65) to help locate their positions. Use your hands to sense over the area where the organs lie, taking the time to visit your liver on the upper right quadrant of your belly, your spleen on the left side of the waist and your kidneys along the sides of the spine just above your waist in the back.

Once you have visited the major players inside your body, let your awareness return to your center in a general way. Feel the soft center and its contents. If you are on the floor, begin to roll like a big seal, feeling the luscious fullness of your internal organs as they soften your movements. Imagine that you are "boneless," and experiment with how much you can move through this central initiation alone.

~ INQUIRY ~

Moving with Organ Support

Sit on the floor in a cross-legged position or on a chair if this is more comfortable. First imagine your body as a skeleton and turn to the right, bringing your left hand onto the outside of your right knee and thigh. Use your skeleton to lever your trunk farther around, and notice how far you have been able to twist by making a mental note of the direction of your gaze. Relax and return to a neutral position.

Now take a moment to sense and feel your inner organ body. Breathe into your belly and, without the use of your arms, initiate the rotation of your trunk by rolling the abdominal organs to the right. As you breathe in, center your attention a little higher in the trunk and roll the liver and stomach to the right as you exhale. Work your way up the body in this way, refining your alignment by sensing the position of the brain and spinal cord. Now bring your left arm around to the outside of your right knee and use your arm to *guide* but not to dictate the twist. Make a mental note of how far you turned this time by noticing where your gaze falls. Did you go farther? If so, can you describe the difference between moving with and without the central initiation of your organs?

Now experiment with a few yoga *asanas* that you already know. Compare what it feels like to move with and without the underlying support of the organs. How does moving from your inner body change the way you feel in the *asanas*? Does it change the way you perceive yourself?

The System in Practice

∽ When you enter a yoga *asana,* pause before making any adjustments to your position. Instead of adjusting from your outer frame, can you initiate the movement from the underlying organs?

∽ Useful organ connections:
  • The centers of the thighs connect to your large intestine on both sides (see Figure 34).
  • Heart and lungs support the arms (see Figure 32).
  • The digestive tract is the frontal support for your spine (see Figure 33).
  • The liver, stomach, and pancreas offer central support for your torso.
  • The line from the kidneys to the bladder connected by the ureters establishes spatial integrity between your rib cage, lower back, and pelvis.

∽ To stimulate your organs you can hum or sound into them. Allow yourself to make sound as you practice.

The Neuroendocrine System

Key Attributes: internal stillness, energetic charge, surges or explosions of chaos/balance, quickness, lightness, effortlessness, radiance, spatial intent

Structure and Qualities: Running through the central channel of the body lie a series of powerfully charged endocrine glands (Figure 35b). These charged points secrete hormones directly into the bloodstream, some at such lightning speeds as to catapult the body into action in seconds. The glands work in intimate concert with one another and with the electrical nervous system to orchestrate the chemical balance of the body. Although relatively small compared to the organs and muscles, the glands have far-reaching effects upon every physiological function of the body. If even one gland produces too much or too little of its elixir, the body can be thrown into a state of complete chaos, impairing the function of all body systems.

Just as the chakras appear to be spinning vortices of energy that lie in a vertical line along our torsos, with each specializing in a different aspect of our physical, emotional, and mental experience,[9] the glands appear to exert both physiological and psychic effects.

A brief mention should be made here about the *chakras,* an energetic system that is given great emphasis in some yogic traditions. The number of chakras ranges, depending on one's source, from three to twenty-three, frequently with major discord between sources on the exact location of each. The seven most well known chakras are the root, sacral, navel, heart, throat, brow, and crown, respectively called in Sanskrit the *Muladhara, Svadhisthana, Manipura, Anahata, Vishudda, Ajna,* and *Sahasrara* centers. Each is symbolically corresponded with specific colors, symbols, sounds, deities, and anatomical sites, and are thought to affect the forces behind functions such as smelling, tasting, seeing, touching, hearing, and perceiving. While there is little agreement on specifics, almost all sources do agree that the chakras function as focal points for the reception and transmission of psychophysical energies.

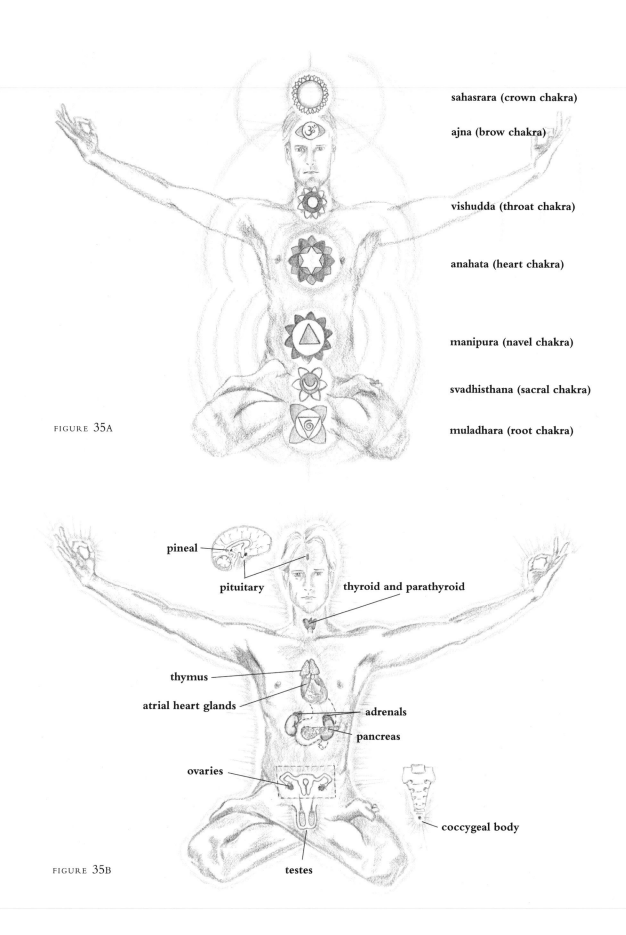

FIGURE 35A

sahasrara (crown chakra)

ajna (brow chakra)

vishudda (throat chakra)

anahata (heart chakra)

manipura (navel chakra)

svadhisthana (sacral chakra)

muladhara (root chakra)

FIGURE 35B

pineal

pituitary

thyroid and parathyroid

thymus

atrial heart glands

adrenals

pancreas

ovaries

coccygeal body

testes

While it would be incorrect to say that the glands of the body are the same as the chakras, there does appear to be a strong relationship between these two systems. The location of the seven major chakras overlaps with that of the glands. It is possible that the two exist on different energetic frequencies, with the chakras acting as the subtle energetic force behind the action of the glands as well as other physiological and psychic functions.

Whether you subscribe to the existence of the chakras is not important. It is always easier to move from the concrete to the subtle, and thus the following inquiries begin with a focus on the glands. Just as you can become more attuned to the tension or relaxation in your muscles, it is possible to tune in to the state of the glands and, by sensitizing yourself to their location, function, and energetic qualities, to engage their support. While this work may seem subtle and even esoteric, we unconsciously notice the presence of the glands in others all the time. We notice certain people stand out when they walk into a room, emanating a glowing charisma or striking presence. Others catch our attention through the vital quickness, agility, and assertiveness of their movement, the sparkle behind their eyes, and the bell-like quality of their voices. When we observe experienced yoga practitioners, the body seems to expand beyond its physical dimensions and their movements are light and agile with clear spatial intent. Even while sitting in quiet meditation some people emanate a potency that even laypeople would find glaringly obvious. While some people naturally have this kind of pizzazz, others need to cultivate the expression of the glands. This expression can be directed outward in dynamic action or inward for containment and rejuvenation.

The chart below will help you locate your glands and gives a list of some of the major physiological functions of each. Once you have read the chart, the inquiry that follows can be used as a template for working with each gland.

THE NEUROENDOCRINE SYSTEM

GLAND OR BODY: Coccygeal Body[10]
DESCRIPTION AND LOCATION: A tiny, irregular, oval-shaped cluster of cells situated at the tip of the coccyx. The coccygeal body is richly supplied with blood vessels and nerve tissue, suggesting it is more than a benign structure.
FUNCTION: Not known.
POSSIBLE CHAKRA CONNECTION: The root chakra, *Muladhara* ("root support"), is associated with the earth element and the lower limbs.

GLAND OR BODY: Sex Glands (Women)
DESCRIPTION AND LOCATION: In women the two almond-shaped ovaries are located roughly in the central pelvic cavity, midway between the navel and the pubis and about a thumb's distance from the midline on each side. Their exact position varies considerably from individual to individual.
FUNCTION: Egg production and reproduction. Secretes estrogens and progesterone, which stimulates and maintains sexual characteristics. Influences behavior.
POSSIBLE CHAKRA CONNECTION: *Svadhishthana* ("own-base") chakra is associated with the water element and sexual energy.

GLAND OR BODY: Sex Glands (Men)

DESCRIPTION AND LOCATION: The two testes, each roughly egg-shaped, are suspended in the scrotum by the spermatic cords. Many men feel a secondary energetic point for the testes in the pelvic cavity (the location of the testes before their descent through the inguinal canal) at roughly the same location as the ovaries.

FUNCTION: Sperm production, storage, and reproduction. The secretion of androgens, testosterone, and androsterone stimulate and maintain sexual characteristics. Influences behavior.

POSSIBLE CHAKRA CONNECTION: *Svadhishthana* ("own-base") chakra is associated with the water element and sexual energy.

GLAND OR BODY: Adrenal Glands

DESCRIPTION AND LOCATION: The two cone-shaped adrenal glands sit on top of the kidneys at about the level of the eleventh and twelfth ribs (slightly above your waist), underneath the diaphragm and behind the muscles of the back.

FUNCTION: The *medulla,* or central portion, of the adrenal glands activates the "fight-or-flight" response through the action of epinephrine (Adrenalin) and norepinephrine. These increase blood pressure and respiration rate, and mobilize muscles for action while simultaneously slowing digestive processes. The *cortex,* or outer portion, is responsible for the production of steroidal hormones and small quantities of androgens and estrogens, which respectively have masculinizing or feminizing effects.

POSSIBLE CHAKRA CONNECTION: *Manipura,* or navel chakra, is associated with the fire element and personal power.

GLAND OR BODY: Pancreas

DESCRIPTION AND LOCATION: The pancreas is a six-inch-long tongue-shaped gland. The hammer-shaped head of the gland snuggles into the duodenum, and the body travels upward and backward to the left, with the tail touching the spleen. Placing one hand slightly above the navel and the other around the left side of the waist roughly describes the position of the gland from head to tail respectively.

FUNCTION: The gland has both endocrine and exocrine functions, with the islets of Langerhans producing insulin and glucagon. Insulin lowers the blood sugar levels by increasing the transport of glucose across cell membranes (especially those of the liver and muscle cells) and is thus essential for energy abundance. Glucagon raises the blood sugar level. The gland's exocrine cells produce about a liter of pancreatic enzymes, which are delivered to the duodenum via ducts for digestion of food.

POSSIBLE CHAKRA CONNECTION: *Manipura* ("jewel-city") chakra is associated with the fire element, the solar plexus, and the main storage center for *prana,* or life-force energy.

GLAND OR BODY: Heart

DESCRIPTION AND LOCATION: The atrial heart muscle has been shown to secrete hormones that regulate body fluids, among other functions.[11]

FUNCTION: Atrial Natriuretic Factor (ANF) is an amino acid polypeptide synthesized by cardiac muscle tissue and secreted into the bloodstream. Stretch of the atrial muscle is the primary stimulus for release of ANF.

POSSIBLE CHAKRA CONNECTION: *Anahata,* or heart chakra, is associated with the air element, the cardiac plexus, and love of others.

GLAND OR BODY: Thymus Gland

DESCRIPTION AND LOCATION: The thymus is a double-lobed butterfly-shaped gland about two inches in length and width in adults. It lies directly behind the upper sternum, on top of the heart. The thymus is conspicuous in infants and reaches its maximum size of about 40 grams at puberty. After puberty, it begins to decrease in size, atrophying in some people to no more than a pad of fat and connective tissue.

FUNCTION: The thymus is essential for the development of immunity. One theory for the rapid atrophy of the thymus after puberty is that the same hormones that bring about puberty also stimulate the migration of the thymus cells to other sites such as the lymph nodes, creating a more global defense mechanism for disease.

POSSIBLE CHAKRA CONNECTIONS: *Anahata,* or heart chakra, is associated with the air element, the sense of touch, the capacity for feeling and compassion for others.

THE NEUROENDOCRINE SYSTEM *(continued)*

GLAND OR BODY: Thyroid Gland

DESCRIPTION AND LOCATION: The thyroid gland is a butterfly-shaped two-lobed gland situated just below the larynx and the thyroid cartilage and on and around the trachea at the base of the neck. The gland weighs about 1 ounce and has a rich blood supply.

FUNCTION: The thyroid's secretions are primarily controlled by thyroid-stimulating hormone secreted by the anterior pituitary gland. The thyroid produces thyroxine and triiodothyronine, which together have a profound effect on the metabolic rate of the body. The thyroid also increases the rates of secretions of most other endocrine glands and secretes calcitonin, which regulates calcium metabolism.

POSSIBLE CHAKRA CONNECTION: *Vishuddha,* or throat chakra, is associated with the ether element, the auditory sense, self-expression, energy, and endurance.

GLAND OR BODY: Parathyroid Glands

DESCRIPTION AND LOCATION: Four small button-shaped discs embedded in the back of the thyroid gland, with one behind each of the upper and lower poles of the thyroid.

FUNCTION: The parathyroid glands secrete parathormone, which controls the calcium levels in the blood as well as the concentration of phosphate in the body. It does this by affecting the absorption of calcium through the intestines, the excretion of calcium from the kidneys, and the release of calcium from the bones.

POSSIBLE CHAKRA CONNECTION: *Vishuddha,* or throat chakra, is associated with the ether element, the auditory sense, self-expression, energy, and endurance.

GLAND OR BODY: Pituitary Gland

DESCRIPTION AND LOCATION: The pituitary is a small pea-sized gland that is connected by a stalk to the hypothalamus. It lies in a tiny depression called the *sella tursica,* or Turk's saddle, in the sphenoid bone, just behind the top of the nasal cavity and slightly in front of the midline of the head. The anterior pituitary is controlled by nerve fibers originating in the hypothalamus, and the posterior pituitary is controlled by hormones secreted by the hypothalamus itself.

FUNCTION: The hypothalamus receives signals and information from the nervous system about the well-being of the body, and this information then determines the secretions of the pituitary gland. The pituitary secretes six very important hormones that promote growth and affect metabolic functions throughout the body. Its actions affect the thyroid, adrenal, and sex glands; regulate the water levels in the body; and induce labor and milk production.

POSSIBLE CHAKRA CONNECTION: *Ajna,* or third-eye chakra, is associated with the processing of sensory input, intuition, telepathic communication, and the ability to meditate.

GLAND OR BODY: Pineal Gland

DESCRIPTION AND LOCATION: The pineal gland is a reddish-gray conical-shaped gland that is located slightly behind and above the pituitary gland, above the midbrain. Comparative anatomists believe it to be a vestigial remnant of the "third eye" present at the back of the head in some reptiles.

FUNCTION: The ancient yogis believed that the pineal gland secreted an ambrosial nectar essential for longevity, and it was thought that this structure was related to the "third eye," or *Ajna* chakra. As such the pineal gland was associated with the ability to "see within," allowing entrance to a pure intuitive perception. Although it is still couched in mystery, modern scientists are finding that the pineal gland is affected by exposure to light, which appears to regulate rhythms of fertility and sexual activity. The pineal gland also secretes *melatonin* and other similar substances, which inhibit the secretions of certain sex hormones.

POSSIBLE CHAKRA CONNECTIONS: *Ajna,* or third-eye chakra, is associated with the processing of sensory input, intuition, telepathic communication, and the ability to meditate.

～ INQUIRY ～

The Glandular Body

Once you have spent some time familiarizing yourself with each of the glands, begin to sense them as a relational system, feeling for the supportive and counter-balancing connections between them.

Stand in a comfortable position. Depending on the time you have available, you can choose to work with one gland each session (perhaps at the beginning of your practice) or you can work sequentially from the tail up to the head. The following is a template for guiding your inquiry:

1. Begin by visualizing the shape and location of the gland. Placing your hands on the external markings that correspond to the gland's position can be helpful. Imagine each gland as a sparkling star inside the body, full of potential.

2. Sense for areas of increased "charge" in and around the gland.

3. Breathe into the gland, imagining that as you breathe in, the gland glows, and as you breathe out, the gland dims. Some people find it helpful to sound into their glands or to use a staccato "hissing" breath to vibrate the gland. Place your tongue behind the back of your front teeth and breathe out, keeping the teeth lightly clenched.

4. Initiate your movement from the gland, noticing how this affects the quality of your movement. Sense how the gland acts to support other structures such as the pelvic floor and sacrum or the arms. Don't be afraid to let the movement take you into space.

5. Come back to your original standing position, feeling the latent potential of the gland when contained in stillness.

～ INQUIRY ～

Glandular Support in Asana *Practice*

Practice any *asana* you know well. Or, if you are a beginner, try the Horseman's Pose on page 96. Once you feel secure in your position and have established the underlying organ support for the movement, close your eyes and imagine the glands in your body as a series of shimmering stars or planets, each hovering in relationship to the others. The pituitary and pineal glands in the head, the thyroid and parathyroid in the throat, the thymus and heart in the chest, the pancreas and adrenals in the abdomen and back, and the sex glands and coccygeal body in the

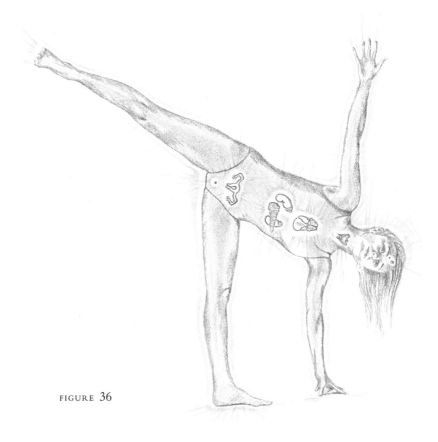

FIGURE 36

pelvis (Figure 36). Depending on the position you have chosen, feel where you need extra support, lift, extension, or reach, and begin to amplify the glands that reside in those areas. Imagine the gland brightening and suffusing the surrounding tissue with such force that the light of the gland expands to meet the surface of the skin and beyond. For instance, if you are extending your leg in a standing posture, explore the connection between your sex glands and the strong anchoring action of the leg to the earth. Or, if the arms are extended, feel for the underlying support from the thymus and heart bodies. Notice how as you engage the support of one gland, you may sense others becoming more dominant as they support or offer counterbalance. Allow the *asana* to reach a place of resolution. When you are finished, pause for a few moments to observe the effects of your practice.

SUMMARY

Engaging the Whole Body

In a democratic body every member in the community gets a chance to express itself and to offer its special contribution. Imagine what it would be like to go to a meeting where a few people dominated all the discussions. These loudmouths would prevent softer-spoken folks with no less important ideas from being heard. Eventually the entire community would be out of balance as a result. Then imagine what it would be like to live in a community where everyone was not only allowed but encouraged to share ideas, perceptions, and insights. Obviously the naturally outspoken would have to tone down a little, and the shy wallflowers would have to be coaxed out of silence. As you have worked your way through the previous inquiries, you have been intentionally shaping a more harmonious body community by encouraging different body systems to speak their mind.

As you progress to learning the yoga *asanas,* you'll now be able to draw upon and modulate the various systems as you need their support. This is rather like adjusting the knobs on your stereo for each new piece of music. In some postures you'll find you need to "turn up the volume" of some systems, while turning down the volume of others. In one *asana* you may find you need strong support and activation of your musculoskeletal system together with the vibrant charge of your glandular system. Other *asanas* like the twists may require greater mobilization of your internal organs. To do flowing sequences of postures, you'll need to bring in the unifying action of your fluids. When you feel lethargic and heavy, you'll be able to draw upon the energizing glands. And, most important, whenever you feel you are losing a sense of center you can descend into the cellular substratum of yourself for insight, rest, and recuperation.

Our individual constitutional nature largely determines our proclivities and thus our tendencies to live in some aspects of our bodies more than others. The purpose of yoga practice is not to change our inherent nature but to expand our choices so that our habit patterns do not create imbalances and limit our growth. Becoming a "broad-spectrum" person not only allows one to operate in the world with greater skill, it also enables one to see and relate to others who are different with welcoming acceptance.

Return
Return the Mind to Original Silence: Developing Clear Perception

Clear inner perception allows us to see ourselves as we truly are.

This last principle acts as an umbrella for all others that have preceded it.

Return. This is the purpose of all spiritual practices. To what do we return? If you look at the sky what you tend to notice is the objects in it—the passing birds or the changing clouds. The ordinary or habitual mind has a tendency to fixate and follow these transient forms without noticing the unchanging and ever present canvas of the sky. When we bring our awareness to rest upon this canvas, we find that it is still, luminous, and silent. A mind filled with such awareness has become awakened to its true nature.

If we wish to practice from the guidance of this silent and clear mind, we must learn to differentiate it from the ordinary workings of our habitual mind. In other words, we must learn to see the sky and to focus our attention on this unchanging background. In contrast, a mind guided by the fickle nature of habitual thinking, in constant obsessive activity, is one that is ungrounded, and the thoughts and actions that flow from such a mind will be equally ungrounded. The challenge in yoga is first to awaken this clear vision in the hothouse conditions of formal practice and then to sustain it under all conditions in our everyday lives. Then when we act in the world, whether it be in regard to a decision or a word spoken, our actions can be based upon and guided by this silent, clear awareness.

This clarity is not something we achieve as a one-off deal but is a state of presence that must be continually renewed through our commitment to practice. Yoga practice is the means and end to achieving clear perception. The paradox of developing this clear perception is that the best way to know is "not to know." Most of what we think we know is conditioned through our past and through the dictates of our own expectations. When we enter a place of "not knowing," we clear the slate of the mind and simply listen in an open way. We let the mind become like the sky—open and unbroken. Not knowing is different from being ignorant. Consciously not knowing is an opening of our intelligence to perceive those possibilities outside the realm of the conditioned mind. By voluntarily removing the walls around the small compound of what we think we know, we can avail ourselves of a fresh awareness. We can achieve this by learning to listen for inner guidance without suppressing, editing, and remodeling the information we receive to fit with what we currently know, or how we wish things to be. The answers to some of our deepest questions lie *in the spaces in between what we know.*

Traditionally yogis have used an awareness of the breath as a means to bring about this meditative state. Because the breath is always present, we can use it as a means of anchoring the mind in that which is constant, in the same way that we might anchor the mind by looking out and letting the sky fill our entire being. In this way we can start to tap into our deeper intuitions and insights. While it is true that self-reflection helps us to act with clarity, it is not spiritual insurance against difficulty in our lives. Developing inner perception does not answer all our questions but helps us to have the inner strength to live with the mystery of our questions.

The reason why it is so important to know how to connect with this core level of yourself is that it is only through self-reflection that you can know the nature of the authentic self. If your yoga practice is driven by your ideas, concepts, ambition, or insecurities, it is unlikely that your practice will bring inner balance, and even possible that it will contribute to more unhappiness in your life. When you act from the vantage point of your authentic self, you will find yourself making choices that are good for you (and usually good for those around you as well).

Hatha yoga practice with its vast repertoire of movement expressions provides us with a veritable jungle gym to watch our reactions and responses to difficulty and challenge. Can we stay anchored in the silent mind regardless of where we find ourselves? What makes yoga yoga and not merely stretching or calisthenics is this mindful embodiment.

Sitting Meditation: Anchoring the Mind in Silence

Sit in a comfortable position in your chair or on the floor with the support of a cushion. Divide your listening process into increments. Each breath cycle represents one increment of time. Breathe in, breathe out. As you breathe in and out, you will undoubtedly also notice sensations, feelings, images, thoughts arising like clouds passing over the sky of your mind. Within the increment of one breath cycle acknowledge the content of these passing forms without becoming fixated upon them, and return to your breath. In the beginning you will notice how extraordinarily difficult it is to return the mind to its original silence. While you are sitting, your mind may be busy gallivanting back and forth from past to future imagined events—elaborating, dramatizing, and catastrophizing as it goes, completely oblivious to the reality of the situation, which is . . . that you are sitting. In order to know how you are right now, you have to come back into your body, sitting still, breathing. All you need do is remind yourself that you are actually sitting still, sensing and feeling the breath. Mentally whisper, "I am sitting still breathing." You need not suppress the actions of your mind, only continually re-mind yourself of the reality of the moment. Breath by breath, you will find yourself descending from this busy cacophony of imaginings into the quiet substrate of yourself. At first these moments will be brief, interrupted by loud imaginings dashing luringly across the screen of your mind. When new to this practice, the beginner will become distraught and frustrated. Don't give up! Your mind has not become suddenly more busy and chaotic—you have simply begun to notice what has been happening all along. Consider this revelation good news and a sign that you are making progress rather than a sign of failure. After some practice, the quiet substrate will become your more dominant experience.

As you become more adept with this practice you can shift your awareness from the breath itself, which although relatively constant is changing and moving, to the mother of the breath. That is, from where does this breath arise and to what does it return? You will begin to notice that the breath is arising out of a silent ground and dissolving back into the same silent ground. When the mind has been prepared through consistent and sincere practice, it will naturally begin to settle itself to focus on the silent original source of the breath. This is not a state that can be forced but one that occurs naturally and spontaneously as the mind begins to see things as they really are.

Spend at least five minutes, preferably at the beginning of your practice, to anchor your mind in silence. Toward the end of your sitting, sense and feel into yourself, asking the question, "What do I need today to bring balance?"

The Baseline Beginning, the Check-in Finish

Before you begin any movement or practice do a "baseline" glance through your body. At the beginning of your practice notice what you have brought with you to the mat that day. Do you feel tired and listless, or rested and energized? Is your mind calm and relaxed, or agitated and tense? Is there any area of the body that is sore or uncomfortable? Is there any organic process that doesn't seem to be functioning well? Headache or constipation are a couple of examples. As you grow in your practice and expand your repertoire, this baseline information will give you invaluable clues as to which poses and practices to do that day to bring balance to your system.

While you are practicing, notice the moment-to-moment changes in your body-mind state, and when you have completed each *asana,* do a "check-in." Do you feel any different from when you began? If you had a headache before doing a forward bend, is it the same, worse, alleviated, or entirely gone after practicing the *asana?* Then at the end of the practice, check in once again to appreciate the overall effects of your session. Do you feel more balanced and relaxed, or did the practice distress or tire you in some way? If you began the session feeling mentally agitated, it is valuable to make note of a change toward clarity and calm as a result of your practice. Noticing these changes can act as powerful motivation to renew your commitment to practice each day. This is why it is so important to practice in a way that leaves you feeling energized, relaxed, and positive rather than finishing your practice tired, tense, and disappointed. If you feel great as a result of your practice, you will eagerly want to return to the mat the next day. It is also why it is so essential to cultivate an inner reference system so your practice meets *your* needs rather than being driven by the dictates of others or even by yoga tradition itself. If you practice to go as far as the person next to you, or to look like the picture in the book, or to achieve difficult postures out of ambition, this is a sure recipe for creating frustration, disappointment, and injury. Checking in with yourself can also help you to identify postures and practices that irritate you and to avoid or modify these in future sessions.

The Principle in Practice

～ The practice is for you; you are not a sacrificial victim to the practice. Therefore, modify the practice to suit your needs and individual constitution.

～ If you get confused or are unsure of yourself in an *asana,* pause, breathe out, relax, and wait for inner guidance.

～ You can receive guidance only when you are calm and receptive. Anger and impatience prevent you from understanding both the cause of your difficulties and possible solutions to your problem. Resist the temptation to become ungrounded because of difficulty.

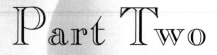

Part Two
~
The Yoga Asanas

III
The Standing Postures

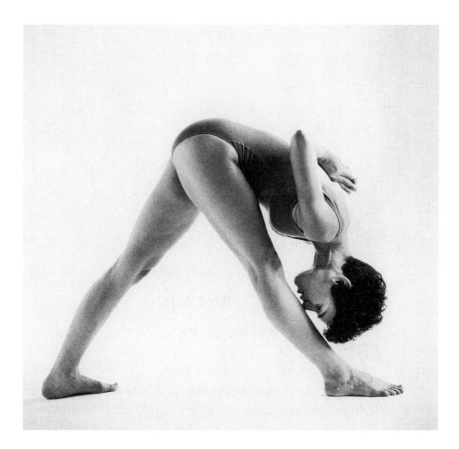

INTRODUCTION

How to Practice the *Asanas*

*T*he following chapters have been organized into families of similar movements. In the beginning of your practice it can be helpful to work progressively through these movements as a way of familiarizing yourself with the skills
needed to practice these *asanas* and to feel more clearly their effects on you. In a
well-balanced practice, however, you would not do twenty backbends in succession, or practice only forward bends. You would practice many different types of
movements sequenced in such a way as to create a feeling of well-being and
balance. In Part Three, you'll find a number of tried-and-true practice sequences
that you can use as guidelines for your own practice. They are best used once you
have a basic familiarity with the *asanas.*

USING THE CHART GUIDES

Cautions

Before you begin practicing each *asana* glance through the chart guide to check
whether this *asana* is suitable for you. Those *asanas* with the ☺ symbol generally

have few contraindications and are user-friendly for most people. I have tried to be conservative in assessing those poses that may be unsuitable for people with particular injuries or health conditions. At the same time, I am acutely aware of how many times students have come for private lessons or group classes with a list of things they "cannot do" only to discover that these same movements are healing for their condition when practiced correctly or modified. While you should heed the advice of your trusted health practitioner, I heartily encourage you also to listen to your own perceptions. If you are recovering from an injury, it is helpful to avoid movements you know aggravate your condition; when you do venture forth to practice these movements again, do 50 percent of what you normally do (in terms of how far you go and how long you stay), and then wait twenty-four hours to see if there are any negative repercussions. Then gradually increase the intensity unless your body tells you otherwise. Difficulties with the more advanced postures such as the Headstand and Shoulder Stand are best addressed with the help of an experienced teacher.

Finally, the "Having Trouble?" section is designed to anticipate the most common problems encountered when practicing an *asana*. It is intended to be a more personal coaching aid. Refer to it often for helpful hints on self-correction.

PRENATAL CONSIDERATIONS

The prenatal symbol, ⊕, will be shaded over the trimester(s) in which the *asana* can be practiced. Experience varies greatly from woman to woman, and if you feel uncomfortable in an *asana,* this is the only guide you need to stop practicing a posture during your pregnancy. If you have complications with your pregnancy, the guidelines given may not be accurate, and you should proceed only with an okay from your health practitioner and work only with an experienced yoga teacher who can give you the one-on-one attention you will need. There are certain things a pregnant woman should be aware of, and I will mention them here in detail as they will appear in abbreviated form in the chart.

In the first trimester of pregnancy many women feel extreme fatigue. Because you may not be "showing" your pregnancy, others may be less sympathetic to your condition at this time. It is therefore even more important that you take care to rest, and if active yoga practices feel too demanding, pamper yourself in one of the many restorative postures in Chapter 7.

After the first trimester you should avoid lying flat on your back. In this position the weight of the baby can press on the inferior vena cava, which is the major blood vessel that returns blood from the lower extremities to your heart. This can prevent blood from returning to the heart and reduce the oxygen supply both to you and your baby. All normally supine postures should be elevated until the back is at an angle steep enough to prevent this pressure against the vein.

During pregnancy the body is literally flooded with hormones that increase the elasticity of the ligaments (the tissues that connect bone to bone where joints meet). Because your connective tissue is offering less support at this time, you should avoid extreme stretching positions, especially those done passively without the support of your muscles. Overstretching ligaments can cause permanent instability in joints such as the sacroiliac. Also, the muscles that support the pelvic floor and the abdominal muscles are already under considerable pressure—this is not a good time to stretch them farther! Long stays in wide-stance standing postures and practicing deep back bends can make postnatal recovery of muscle tone considerably more challenging.

ESSENTIAL SKILLS

Begin each chapter by working through the "Essential Skills" section, which introduces you to the core motif movement at the heart of the other postures. In Chapter 2 you learned about universal movement principles that you can apply to all yoga *asanas*; the essential skills are more detailed, specific skills that you'll need to practice each group of *asanas* with ease and enjoyment. Don't be tempted to skip this section, because the foundation you build here will save you lots of time and frustration later. Because these skills and movements are true for almost all the *asanas* in this family, by mastering them you'll be able to apply them to every posture you practice in this section. In doing so you will no longer be bound to follow a tedious step-by-step list of instructions for each pose. And, if you are having a problem, it's likely you'll be able to backtrack to one or more of these supporting movements.

The inquiries in this section are designed not only to help you learn new skills but also to enable you to identify your normally unconscious body habits. You can be sure that whatever habits you have in simple positions like standing or sitting will consistently carry through into the more complex movements. That is, if you walk with a limp you will run with it, too. By noticing habits such as clenching your toes, holding your breath, or hyperextending your back, you'll be able to put together a personal checklist that you can use when you practice alone. Foreknowledge of your own tendencies will enable you to anticipate your most likely misalignments. You can use this checklist to remind yourself frequently to relax your toes, breathe out, or soften your lower back. This will allow you to be more skillful when practicing alone at home.

INCORPORATING THE SEVEN MOVING PRINCIPLES

Although all seven movement principles are in play in every *asana,* I've emphasized those that are particularly helpful at the beginning of each chapter. Take a moment to tweak your memory by glancing through just one of these principles at the beginning of your practice. You can use this principle as the thread for the day's practice. For instance, if the principle is about learning to yield to the earth, you can focus your awareness on giving your weight through your feet and legs in all the standing postures, experimenting until you find just the right degree of tension. If the principle is about letting the breath oscillate the body, you can explore what that means for you in your arms, legs, and spine, returning again and again to the central theme of the principle just as a composer might return to a melodic theme.

If you are experiencing difficulty in a posture, consider which principle may help you. If you feel stiff and segmented, could more awareness of your body as a fluid medium help you feel ease and integration? You might be experiencing discomfort in your back, and this will be a clue to revise and focus on the essential elongation of your spine. Whenever you are having trouble, resist the temptation to get flustered or irritated. Stay calm and focused, and the next step will become clear to you. If you think your problem requires the help of someone more knowledgeable and experienced, make a note to bring these issues up with your yoga teacher. Whenever possible, however, cultivate self-sufficiency and resourcefulness. If you have a question, it is because you are in the process of answering it. While a skilled teacher can help you move more swiftly through your process, learning through direct exploration and discovery can never be entirely bypassed.

The Standing Postures

The standing postures teach us to stand on our own two feet. They invigorate, heat, and strengthen the entire body, increasing our circulation and stamina. The emphasis in this group of *asanas* is on establishing a firm base of support through the legs so that the spine can be relaxed, light, and free. When the arms and legs are weak, unstable, or poorly integrated, the spine becomes tense and overworked, becoming the *supporting* rather than the *supported* structure.

The standing postures teach us to conduct force through the body so that we become clear conduits between heaven and earth. As we give our weight to the earth there is a rebounding upward force that rises through the legs. If our feet, ankles, knees, and hips are aligned well, we can direct this rebounding force into the spine. The standing postures can thus indirectly affect even serious back problems, because this force can be used to elongate, strengthen, balance, and release the spine. Because the spine is usually in a relatively neutral position, these postures are some of the safest and most effective for correcting spinal imbalances.

Standing postures can be practiced every day and should form the core of a beginner's practice. These postures take the body gently through almost all the possible ranges of motion—forward bending, back bending, side bending, and twisting. This synergistic work conditions the whole body and prepares it for more intense practice.

KEY MOVING PRINCIPLES FOR THE STANDING POSTURES

2. YIELD

Yield to the Earth: Weight and Levity

3. RADIATE

Move from the Inside Out: The Human Starfish

4. CENTER

Maintain the Integrity of the Spine: The Central Axis

ESSENTIAL SKILLS

Standing Well—Mountain Pose (*Tadasana*)

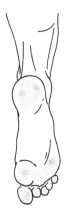

FIGURE 38

～ The Feet: Foundations of Support for the Legs

Your legs mirror everything you do with your feet. The position of your feet and the distribution of weight through them will affect the position, function, and flow of force higher up through your knees, your hips, and even your back. If your feet are clenched and tight, your whole body reflects this tension, too. Because you can see your feet, it is relatively easy to perceive them. Your weight should be equally distributed between the ball and heel of your foot and the inner and outer foot with all the toes spreading to form a wide base of support (Figure 38).

～ INQUIRY ～

Centering the Weight on the Feet

Come to a standing position, *first* noticing your habitual posture. Observe whether you stand with the feet close together or wider than your hips and whether you turn your feet in or out. Do you stand on the heels or the toes, or put more weight through one foot? Check to see whether you contract your toes or collapse your arches. Make a mental note of what you've discovered.

Place your feet hips-width apart with the inner edges of your feet parallel to each other. Now begin to rock your weight forward and back, alternating between placing the weight on the toes and then on the heels. Gradually, over the course of ten breaths, make these oscillations smaller until you feel your weight balanced over the center of each foot. When the weight is balanced over your feet, it will come through the balls of your feet and spread evenly across your heels. The arches will be lifted away from the floor as each toe extends lightly forward. When you feel your weight evenly placed on your feet, lift and spread your toes to widen your base of support even further. In all the postures continually bring your awareness back down into your feet, checking that you are maintaining a balanced distribution of weight through the soles of your feet and between both of your legs.

~ The Pelvis: Foundation of Support for the Spine

Your pelvis is like a beautiful round pot, out of which the tree of your spine grows. If the pot is tipped forward or back or to one side, the tree cannot grow straight. The first thing we learn in standing is how to bring the pelvis into a level, or *neutral,* position that allows the spine to be in a neutral position as well.

~ INQUIRY ~

Centering the Pelvis

Stand in your habitual way and place your fingers on the creases of your groin just underneath your hipbones. Imagine the pelvis as a large bowl filled with water. When your pelvis is in a neutral position, the water will lie level (Figure 39a). Tip your pelvis under so that the water pours out the back of the bowl (Figure 39b). As you do this, notice that the tissue under your fingers has become hard and sinewy, like a guitar string tuned to a high pitch. Now tip your pelvis forward so that the water pours out the front of the bowl (Figure 39c). Notice that the tissue under your fingers has now become like an oversoft mattress. Experiment by tipping the pelvis forward and back, alternating between the too-tight, too-soft sensations under your fingers. Now explore the middle position. When the water in your pelvic bowl is level, you will feel a little end-spring under your fingers. This sensation of slight tension tells that your pelvis is in a neutral position and that you are now standing on your bones, rather than sitting into your lower back or your groin.

Make a note of your personal tendencies. If you sling your pelvis under, your lower back will be too flat (hypolordotic). People who stand like this tend to balance the forward thrust of the hips by hanging the chest behind the line of gravity and thrusting the head forward as a counterbalance (see Figure 39b). If you arch your pelvis forward, your lower back will be too deeply curved (hyperlordotic). People who stand like this tend to thrust the lower ribs and chest forward (see Figure 39c). When you stand with a neutral pelvis, your spine will be long and released and your chest and head will be balanced over your belly (see Figure 39a).

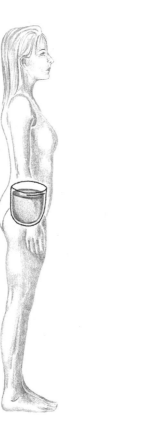

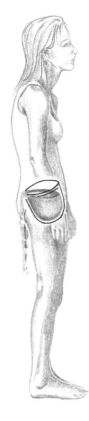

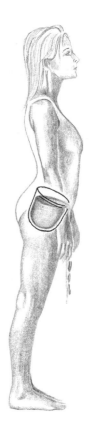

39A. *Normal*   39B. *Hypolordotic (flat lower back)*   39C. *Hyperlordotic (swayback)*

THE PREPARATORY STANCES

All the standing postures begin from one basic stance. Establishing a correct and balanced foundation gives you a stable base from which to move. Keep in mind that all the standing postures are movements that exist in more than one plane. Although the postures may appear flat and two-dimensional in the drawings and photographs, if you try to mimic this you will be forced to move in a very unnatural and stilted manner. As you practice the *asanas* imagine the movements in your mind's eye as sculptural forms, allowing the round curves and natural asymmetries of your body to find their own logic.

~ INQUIRY ~

Preparatory Stance I

Stand with your feet hips-width apart. Extend your arms out to your sides level with your shoulders, and mentally drop a plumb line from your wrists to the floor. Now step your feet wide apart so that your feet are positioned under your wrists.

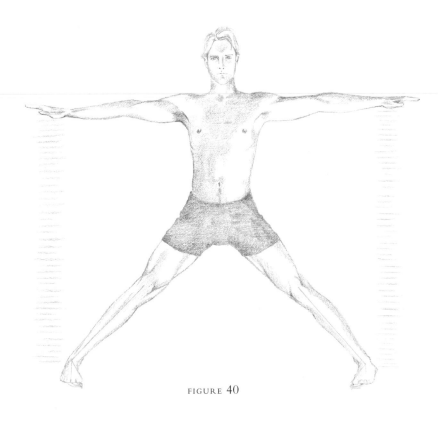

FIGURE 40

Everyone has different body proportions, so this distance is approximate. Turn your feet about 30 degrees inward. This inward rotation will allow your knees to align over your ankles and prevent your feet from slipping apart (Figure 40). Test your position. Bend your knees to check whether your knees track over your feet—if not, you probably need to turn your feet farther inward.

Preparatory Stance II

In most of the standing postures one foot will turn out 90 degrees while the other remains turned inward. Let's try it. Turn your right foot out by pivoting on your heel, spreading your toes, and stretching the foot forward and resting it lightly on the floor. Notice that as you rotate the foot outward the entire leg must rotate outward as well. To do this the left side of your pelvis must move forward so that when you look down, your left hip will be slightly forward of your right hip (Figure 41). This small adjustment makes it easier to keep your entire right leg rotated outward over the right ankle and toe.

Whenever you turn your feet in a particular direction your "knees must obey the feet" so that both the knee and foot are in agreement about where they are going. The pelvis must revolve forward so that this relationship in the legs can be maintained. In Figure 42 (incorrect) the model has tried to keep his hips level, and thus he has forced his front knee to rotate inward. He is also creating unnecessary

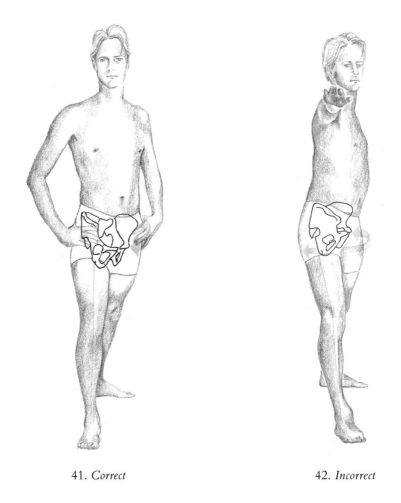

41. *Correct*   42. *Incorrect*

compression in his sacroiliac joints (the joints between the sacrum and the two sides of the pelvis) and lower back. Over time this common error can cause serious back, hip, and knee problems. Whenever you rotate the front leg outward in a standing posture, it is anatomically impossible to keep your pelvis level on both sides. Someone with a very tight groin will have to allow the pelvis to rotate farther forward than a more flexible person, but no one can keep the two sides of the pelvis flush without impairing the function of the hips, knees, and lower back.

Your final check in this posture is to look down to see whether the heel of your right foot aligns with the arch or the inner heel of the back leg. Experiment to see which alignment offers you the greatest stability. You can use a floorboard or a line on the floor as a way to guide you the first time. Now you are ready for the last skill.

THE SITTING BONE TO HEEL CONNECTION

In all human movement there is a powerful connection between the sitting bones of your pelvis and your heels. When you walk, run, or hop on one foot, your body is always trying to find the power line between your feet and the heads of your femurs as a way to stay in balance and for maximum transmission of force from the legs into the torso. Superb runners use this connection to propel themselves forward clearly without wasting energy by veering off the power line.

～ INQUIRY ～

Finding the Sitting Bone to Heel Connection

Take a moment as you are sitting to bring your fingers under your buttocks and feel for the two prominent sitting bones (the *ischial tuberosities*). Bring your feet hips-width apart and place your feet so they are directly under the knees. Now mentally draw a line from the sitting bone of each side of the pelvis to your heels. Press down firmly with the heel of your right foot and feel how this moves force into the right side of your pelvis. Then take your right foot 1 foot farther out to the side so that it is no longer in line with your sitting bone. Press through your foot again. Then bring your right foot to rest beside the inside of your left foot and press again. Can you feel how the transmission of force to your pelvis is not as clear when the heel is outside the line of the sitting bone?

Return to the Preparatory Stance II with your right leg turned out. Look at the heel of your right foot, and mentally draw a line from your heel along the floor underneath you to the other foot. Now bring your right sitting bone forward over this line. If you are unsure, stand on a floorboard, aligning your front heel with your back arch. Once you bring your right sitting bone forward in line with the heel, you will no longer be able to see the right heel when you look down. Slowly bend your right knee, keeping the right sitting bone in line with your right heel. Did you find that you had to let your left hip come forward to do this? When you find this natural power line, your knee will align beautifully over the ankle so that when you look down you can see only your big toe. If you can see all your toes, you have probably moved the sitting bone back and turned the knee inward. Also, when you press back

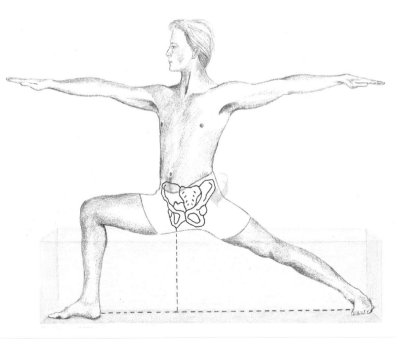

through your right foot, you'll be able to send force clearly through your knee, hip, across the bridge of your pelvis, and all the way into the other leg and foot. Try this for yourself. Push back from your front leg until you can feel a strong connection between your front foot and your back foot (Figure 43).

In Figure 42 you can see the results of losing this power line. As the sitting bone and hip fall behind the line of the heel, the knee turns inward and the arch of the front foot collapses. Because the legs are no longer underneath the torso, the spine has been thrust forward. Now the spine becomes tense as it takes on the *supporting* rather than *supported* role.

FIGURE 43

A NOTE ABOUT THE KNEES

The knee is a hinge joint, but when the leg is bent a slight degree of rotation is possible. This adaptation allows you to make quick changes of direction, as when a soccer player maneuvers a ball, but it also makes the knee vulnerable to injury. In all the standing postures the knees must turn to follow the angle of the foot so that the joint acts as a hinge. When you turn your leg outward in preparation for a standing posture, prevent the kneecap from rotating inward by drawing the muscles above your knee (the quadriceps) gently up as if to make the corners of your knee "smile." This will lift and stabilize the kneecap. It should feel as if the knee is floating up the leg rather than gripping the joint. When this is done correctly, you will not be able to move your patella (kneecap) side to side with your fingers. If you are not sure how to do this, sit on the floor with your legs extended in front of you. Raise one leg an inch off the floor. The action necessary to lift the leg uses the same muscles required to lift the kneecap. *Never* press the kneecap downward or forcefully lift the kneecap, as this will lock the knee and hyperextend the joint, causing strain inside the joint and in the tendons along the back of the leg. Respectful positioning of your knees in all the postures will ensure that you'll keep those handy hinges healthy!

With these three skills under your belt you are ready to begin.

THE STANDING POSTURES

Spinal Rolls

Here's How

Stand in Mountain Pose. Slowly lower your head until your chin is resting on or close to your chest (Figure 44). Open your mouth and take several long, deep, audible sighs through your mouth. Close your eyes, and notice that as you breathe, your head and neck are bobbing up and down on the current of the breath. Once you feel this pulsing action, slowly begin to curl forward, vertebra by vertebra through your spine until you are hanging over your legs. As soon as you begin to bend forward, release your knees, increasing the bend as you fold farther forward. At the bottom of the movement take a few deep breaths, letting your head, spine, and arms hang loosely (Figure 45).

Now begin your ascent. Pressing down through your feet, gradually stack the bones of the spine one over the other, straightening your legs as you come up. Synchronize the movement of the spinal rolls so that your knees are in constant motion—bending slowly as you go down, gradually straightening as you come up. Each time you come up to a standing position, check that your shoulders are released downward, your belly is open and receptive, and your neck is elongated.

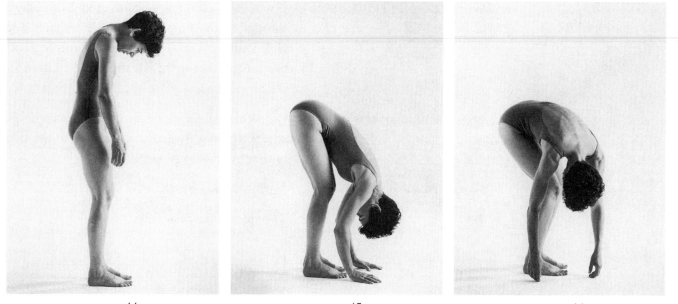

FIGURE 44   FIGURE 45   FIGURE 46

Now look down at your right little toe. You will now do the same movement, except you'll bend on a diagonal to the side. Keep your knees parallel and continue to let your arms drape loosely downward as you fold to the side (Figure 46).

Repeat the Spinal Rolls three times—to the center, left, and right. Each time you roll down, tune in to the sensations in your back. Are there any segments that feel particularly stiff or glued together? Slow down around these segments, using the rocking motion of your breath to gently pry the bones apart.

Variation

On a Chair   If the backs of your legs (the hamstrings) are very stiff or you have spinal problems, you can try the Spinal Rolls while sitting on a chair. This variation is also good when you are at work or traveling, as you can release your back without drawing attention to yourself.

Sit on the edge of your chair with your feet wide apart to form a tripod between your buttocks and legs. In this variation you roll down only to the center, letting your arms drape around the outsides of your thighs. If you wish to intensify the stretch along the backs of your legs, walk your feet out a few inches and release the back forward once more. As you begin each repetition increase the distance between your feet and the chair in 1-inch increments. When you are ready to come up, walk your feet back underneath you, press down through the soles of your feet, and roll up through your spine. If you have a weak back, place your hands on the seat of the chair alongside your hips to support your ascent.

BENEFITS AND EFFECTS   Releases the spine and stretches the hamstrings. Gradually loosens and engages the whole body. Centers the mind.

WHO SHOULDN'T DO THIS POSE	If you have a bulging or herniated disc, flexion through your spine may cause problems. Try Half-Dog Pose (page 97) with the arms high on the wall so that there is a slight indentation in your lower back.
PRENATAL SUGGESTIONS	⊕ Widen the stance if necessary to accommodate your belly. Avoid the spinal rolls to the side as your pregnancy progresses.
HAVING TROUBLE?	My lower back hurts.
TRY ...	*The Chair Variation or Half-Dog Pose*

Horseman's Pose (*Utkatasana*)

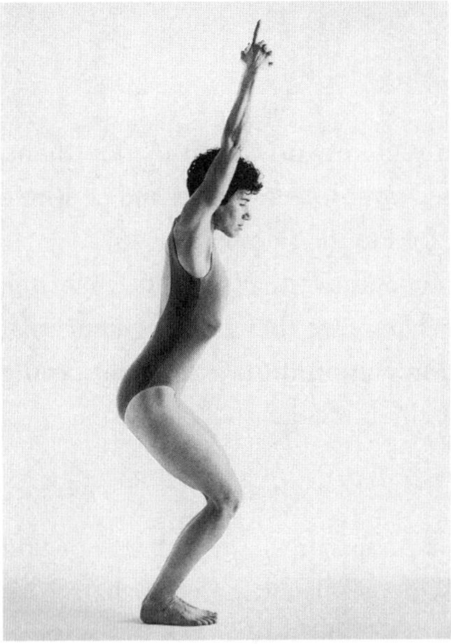

FIGURE 47

Here's How

Stand in Mountain Pose with the inner edges of your feet touching. On an inhalation extend your arms overhead and hook your thumbs. Reaching strongly upward, slowly bend your knees. As you deepen in the position, maintain a clear line from your head through to your tail, using the front of your body to support your back body (Figure 47). Stay here for three to five breaths, and then slowly release, coming back to a standing position.

Horseman's Pose can be added at the beginning of the Sun Salutation (page 125) as an excellent way to increase strength and endurance.

BENEFITS AND EFFECTS	Strengthens the thighs, abdominal muscles, and back. Opens the chest. Warms the body and improves endurance.
WHO SHOULDN'T DO THIS POSE	☺
PRENATAL SUGGESTIONS	⊕
HAVING TROUBLE?	My lower back hurts.
TRY ...	*You are probably allowing your back to sway by releasing your abdominal muscles. Draw the belly in and up to support your back, and deepen the squat further only if you can maintain this frontal support.*

Half-Dog Pose (*Ardha Svanasana*)

Here's How

Stand with your hands shoulders-width apart on a wall. Slowly walk your feet away from the wall, tipping forward from your hips until your spine and legs form a table position. On an inhalation, press your hands into the wall, and as you exhale, reach back through your sitting bones and tail to elongate your spine. Also allow your torso to rise upward slightly as you breathe in and release downward as you breathe out (Figure 48).

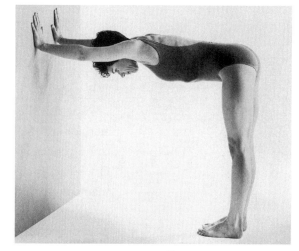

FIGURE 48

In this *asana* make sure that your spine is in a neutral position with all the curves intact (see Figure 14, page 42). You should be able to feel a slight indentation in your lower back. If not, you are flexing forward from your lumbar, which is stressful on your intervertebral disks. To adjust, first try bending your knees and rotating your sitting bones upward. If you are unable to reestablish your lumbar curve (a limitation caused by tight hamstrings), adjust your position by raising your arms up the wall until your back forms one long diagonal line (see Figure 21, page 53). As your legs release, you can gradually work the hands down the wall, all the time moving from the hips while maintaining a neutral position in the spine.

Variations

A: When you are traveling or at work you can use a window ledge, the side of your car, or a chair to support your hands, or you can bend your elbows and perform the posture with your elbows resting on a supporting surface (Figure 49).

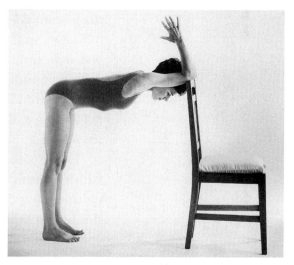

FIGURE 49

B: To loosen tight shoulders, stand a foot away from a wall and slide your elbows up the wall, bringing your hands behind your head with your fingertips touching. Press your armpits toward the wall as you draw the chest toward the wall.

BENEFITS AND EFFECTS	Releases the shoulders, back, and hamstrings. Elongates the spine. Eliminates fatigue and compression in the back muscles.
WHO SHOULDN'T DO THIS POSE	This *asana* is good for all people as long as adjustments are made to ensure neutral spinal curves.
PRENATAL SUGGESTIONS	
HAVING TROUBLE?	I feel tension in my neck and shoulders.

Try . . .

Broaden your shoulders away from your ears by turn-
ing your outer arms downward. Bring your head up so
that your ears are level with your arms and your head
is following the line of your spine.

Triangle Pose (*Trikonasana*)

Here's How

Begin in Preparatory Stance II to the right. As you breathe in, extend your arms out to the sides in line with your shoulders. As you breathe out, slowly begin to tip your pelvis over the right thigh. Imagine your pelvis like the central dial of a clock and your spine as the hand. As you tip sideways, go only as far as you can, maintaining the elongation of your spine from head to tail. When you have gone as far as your legs will comfortably allow, rest your right hand on a block or chair placed next to your ankle (Figure 50), just below the knee, along the shin, or on the floor behind the ankle, depending on your flexibility (Figure 51). As you reach this full position use your breath to focus your attention on the two dynamic actions of the posture. As you breathe in, anchor your legs to the earth, and as you breathe out, allow your spine to elongate from head to tail. With each outgoing breath, widen the span of your arms so the back of the body is broad. Keep your head in a neutral position, and toward the end of your stay in the posture, turn to look up and beyond your left hand. Do this briefly to complete the gesture. After ten breaths, push down through your feet to come up. Now take the *asana* to the left side.

This is one posture in which the principle of navel radiation and the image of the starfish will really help you. In Figure 52 notice that the model has thrust his arm behind him in an attempt to open his chest, but he organizes this around a contracted center that is turning in the opposite direction. Notice how his limbs seem disconnected from the core. To correct this, try practicing the posture while keeping your upper arm resting on your side. First tune in to your breathing, mobilizing your core. Now place your hand on your belly, encour-

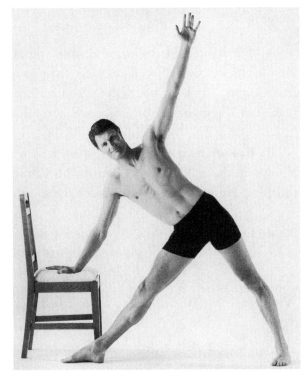

FIGURE 50

aging your belly to turn upward on your exhalation. Once you feel the belly open, move your hand a little higher up the body, working all the way up to the chest, where you can encourage your heart and lungs to turn toward the sky. Once you feel your center has expanded, extend your upper arm again, sensing for the connection between this now open core and your soaring limbs. Let your legs extend down to the earth all the way from the center of your body. With each breath let yourself alternately expand and condense from your center like a starfish.

Variations

Beginners:

～ If you have spinal problems or are very tight through your legs, try placing a block or the seat of a chair underneath your supporting hand (see Figure 50, opposite). Having your hand elevated will reduce the intensity of the movement and prevent you from bearing down on the extended leg with your arm. *You can use the block to adjust your stance in all of the standing postures.*

Advanced:

～ To increase the rotation through the spine, extend your top arm around the back of your body, taking hold of the upper thigh of the extended leg. Use this arm to encourage the spine into a deep twist as you release your upper shoulder back and open your chest. Be careful to elongate the spine as you twist so you do not compress the lower back.

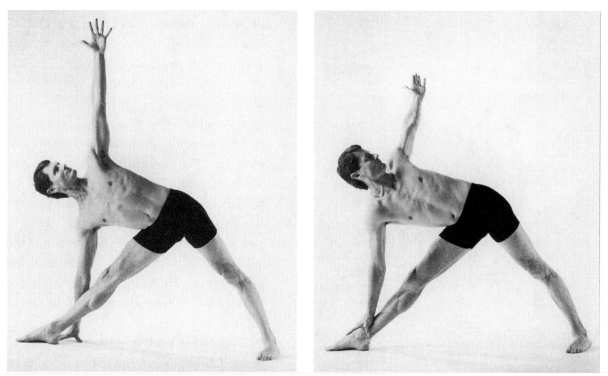

FIGURE 51   FIGURE 52. *Incorrect*

BENEFITS AND EFFECTS

Releases the hips, legs, and the entire spinal column. Opens the sides of the body. Releases the spine.

WHO SHOULDN'T DO THIS POSE

People with posterolateral disc herniation may find the slight twisting action of this posture challenges the back. Raise the hand onto the seat of a chair or block. If there is still pain, come out of the posture.

PRENATAL SUGGESTIONS

Raise your hand onto a block or chair as your pregnancy progresses.

HAVING TROUBLE?

I feel a strong pull on the back of my front knee.

TRY . . .

You are probably collapsing all the weight onto the heel of the front foot. This causes the stretch to be localized at the insertion points of the hamstrings (top of the thigh, back of the knee). Shift your weight forward onto the ball of your foot and maintain this weight distribution as you come into the pose.

Side-Angle Pose (*Parsvakonasana*)

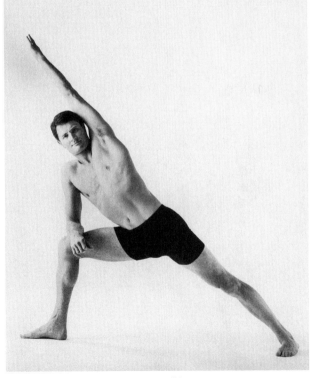

FIGURE 53

Here's How

This *asana* is very similar to Triangle Pose except the stance is wider. Begin in Preparatory Stance II on the right side. Extend your arms to the side on an inhalation, and as you exhale simultaneously tip to the side while bending the right knee. Rest your elbow on the upper thigh, using the elbow to encourage the deep external rotation of your hip (Figure 53). Now is the time to adjust the width of your stance, if necessary. If your knee is extending forward past the line of your ankle, broaden your stance. If you are unable to bring your knee over the ankle, narrow the stance. When the knee lies directly over the ankle and the thigh and shin form a right angle, you will be in the most stable position.

Now press back from your right leg to bring the weight into the left leg. Once you feel the left leg strongly anchored, slowly extend the left arm over your head, by first grazing your fingers to your ear and then straightening the arm. Your body should form one long diagonal line from your back leg through your torso through to your arm. As you become stronger in the legs and more flexible in your hips, you can complete the pose by bringing your right fingertips to rest on the floor behind your foot (Figure 54). Keep your head in a neutral position with your eyes gazing forward for most of your stay in this posture; in the last few breaths turn your head to gaze up toward the arm.

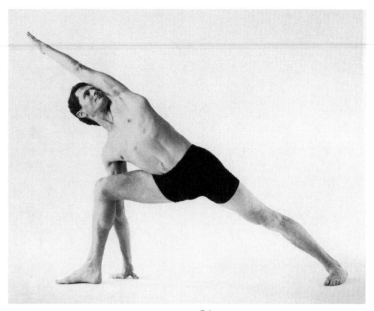

FIGURE 54

The most common error in Side Angle is caused by collapsing the back leg, first by dropping the inner arch of the foot, and then by dropping your knee downward. This puts strain on the back knee and causes your pelvis and lower back to collapse toward the floor (Figure 55). To correct this tendency place the outer edge of your back foot against a wall. Your challenge is to align the lower leg bones with the upper leg bones. Because of their deep angle to the floor, they naturally tend to drop downward. To resist this tendency imagine that you are lifting the sides of your leg up toward the ceiling until the leg bones form one clear line from foot to hip. As you do this, lift the base of your pelvis so that your tail is now pointing toward your back heel. Then let your torso continue this line so that the force from

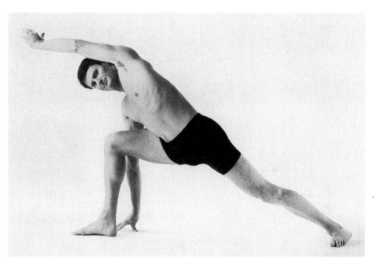

FIGURE 55. *Incorrect*

your back leg is moving clearly into your trunk and spine (see Figure 17, page 50). If you have been accustomed to collapsing through your joints, you may be surprised how much your leg muscles need to work to support this clear alignment. Over time, however, this new way of using yourself will feel light and effortless.

Variation

Advanced: To increase the rotation through the spine, extend your top arm around the back of your body, taking hold of the upper thigh of your extended leg. Use this arm to encourage the spine into a deep twist as you release the shoulder back and open your chest further.

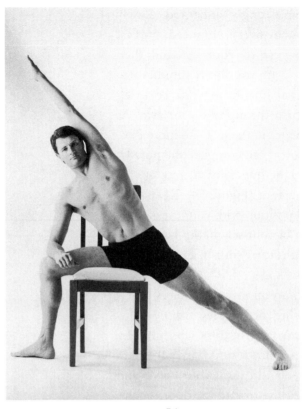

FIGURE 56

BENEFITS AND EFFECTS	Strengthens the legs and releases the hips. Opens the chest and shoulders. Elongates the entire spinal column.
WHO SHOULDN'T DO THIS POSE	☺
PRENATAL SUGGESTIONS	⊕. Practice with the elbow on the thigh, as this gives you more room for your belly. In the early stages of pregnancy when you may feel fatigue, and in the later stages when you should avoid overstretching your pelvic floor, place the seat of a chair underneath the thigh of the front leg (Figure 56). You can use this aid in Warrior Pose II as well.
HAVING TROUBLE?	All my weight seems to be in the front leg.
TRY ...	*Yielding to the earth with the back leg can best be felt if you first bend your knee, letting your weight shift into your back foot. Imagine that your foot is on a sprint block and you are about to propel yourself into the diagonal stretch. To come into the pose, push off and uncoil from the back leg. Whenever you lose the contact of the back foot with the floor, repeat this exercise.*

Warrior Pose II (*Virabhadrasana* II)

Here's How

Begin in Preparatory Stance II on the right side. In this *asana* the front knee bends, but your spine stays suspended in a clear vertical line between your two legs. Take a breath in, extending your arms strongly out to the sides. Let your breath open your heart and lungs so that they can offer their organic support to the outreached arms. On an exhalation, slowly bend your right knee several inches. Without coming up push horizontally back through your right leg until you can feel the weight coming into your back foot. The first time you come into the position, bend the knee in increments, testing at each level that you have maintained equal weight distribution between the two legs. In the full posture your front thigh will be parallel to the floor.

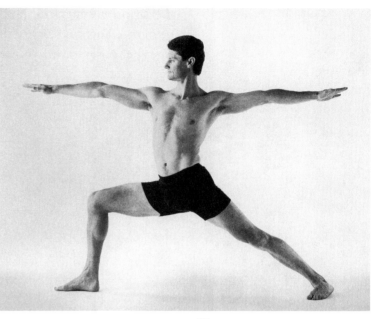

FIGURE 57

Breathe deeply, as this pose requires lots of energy! As you breathe out, imagine yourself expanding from your center, letting all your limbs release away from your belly. Keep the pelvis lightly lifted up off your legs so that your hips will be open and your spine can ascend freely. Turn to gaze toward your right hand and beyond, all the while keeping your spine centered over your pelvis (Figure 57).

BENEFITS AND EFFECTS	Strengthens the legs and increases the flexibility of the hips and groin. Heats the body. Increases stamina and determination.
WHO SHOULDN'T DO THIS POSE	Those with cardiac problems or high blood pressure should approach this pose with caution. Practicing with the arms down by the sides, hands resting on the hips, will reduce strain on the heart.
PRENATAL SUGGESTIONS	Use the chair support as in Side-Angle Pose (Figure 56, page 102) if tired or in the later stage of pregnancy.
HAVING TROUBLE?	My spine leans over my front leg.
TRY . . .	*Reach through your back arm so that your wrist is over your back ankle. If you maintain this relationship, your spine will remain centered.*

Warrior Pose I (*Virabhadrasana* I)

Here's How

Let's work through this posture in a series of variations that are progressively more intense. You can practice them all in succession or alternate in between practicing other poses so that you are gradually moving into the more intense variations as your body warms. Or you can choose the variation that challenges you and concentrate on that one alone.

Start in Preparatory Stance II to the right. Turn your entire body to face your right leg, letting your back heel come off the floor, pivoting the foot to face forward. Let your back knee touch the floor (use a blanket to cushion your knee if necessary), and bring your hands either side of your foot. In this lunge position, focus on allowing your hips to release toward the floor, gradually increasing the opening through the front of the groin. Take ten breaths here. Now bring your hands up onto your thigh, drawing your lower abdomen away from your leg so that your back is upright. Press your

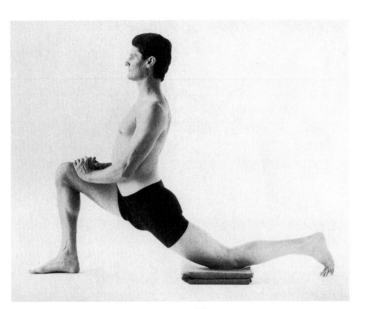

FIGURE 58

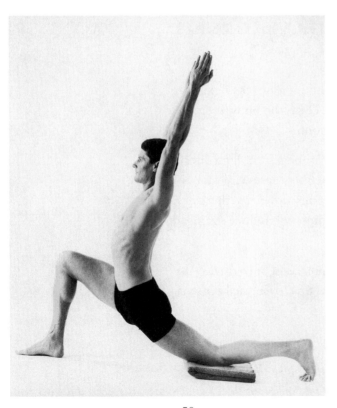

FIGURE 59

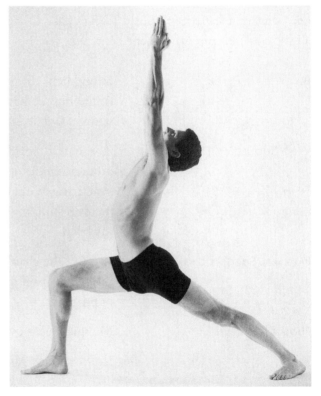

FIGURE 60

hands down against your thigh, raising your chest. You should feel a strong opening throughout your groin and belly (Figure 58). Stay for ten breaths.

Continuing from the previous variation, now extend your arms over your head as you take an inhalation. Focus on lengthening your spine upward and gradually drawing the back into a gentle arc. Do not arch the back so strongly that you feel compression or pain in your lower back. Take five breaths here, each time lifting a little higher into the movement (Figure 59).

For the final position, slowly extend the back heel to straighten the leg, lifting the knee off the floor. Your back heel will now be slightly turned in. If you feel unstable, place your back heel against a wall. Continue to lift up through the arms, interlocking the thumbs and pressing your palms upward. As you lengthen your spine, gradually arc backward, at first keeping your gaze level with the horizon. As you feel more confident of your balance allow your head to release backward in the gesture of completion (Figure 60).

Variations

Beginners: If you have weak legs or unstable balance you can do the final position facing a wall, with your toes touching the wall and your hands at shoulders-height pressing against the wall.

Those with sensitive lower backs: If you have a tendency to compress your lower back, try practicing this posture with the front foot elevated on the seat of a chair. Focus on the upward movement of your spine rather than the back-bending action.

BENEFITS AND EFFECTS	Opens the front of the groin, releasing the deep inner muscles of the pelvis and back. Strengthens the thigh and upper back muscles. Heats and invigorates the body.
WHO SHOULDN'T DO THIS POSE	Those with weak hearts or high blood pressure should not bring the arms over the head. Practice the later variations with your hands on your hips and stay only for a short duration.
PRENATAL SUGGESTIONS	The weight of the abdomen in this position may strain the back, especially in the later stages of pregnancy.
HAVING TROUBLE?	I feel shaky and lose my balance easily.
TRY . . .	*Before you bring your arms off your thigh, push back from your front foot until you can feel the weight coming through your back leg. This will create a base of support from your front leg through your pelvis to your back leg. Keep your gaze level with the horizon.*

Flank Pose (*Parsvottanasana*)

Here's How

In this *asana* the Preparatory Stance is slightly narrower (by about 4 inches), and the back foot turns farther inward so that the pelvis can turn to face the front leg. The easiest way to find the stance is to stand in Mountain Pose with your feet hips-width apart. Imagine that you are standing on a railway track and that as you step your left foot behind you, you want to keep the back foot on the track. If you bring the back foot inside the track, both sitting bones will no longer be in line with your heels and you will feel ungainly in your balance.

From this position place your hands on your hips and slowly bend forward from your hips, keeping your spine long from head to tail. As you bend forward, resist the temptation to swing your right hip off the railway track. This will bring your sitting bone off the line of your right heel and will cause your spine to veer to the left. Go only go as far as you can maintaining the elongation of your spine. Place your fingers on the seat of a chair for support, staying for ten breaths on each side (Figure 61). Focus on broadening the muscles through the backs of the legs. To come up, anchor your weight into your feet and pivot from the hips. Now practice the other side.

If you were comfortable in the previous variation, you are ready to try the classic posture. Stand in Preparatory Stance II with the right leg turned out as above. On an inhalation extend your arms to the sides and bring them behind your back into prayer position (*Namaste*) with the palms pressing together and the fingers facing up toward your neck. If your wrists or shoulders will not allow this, simply clasp the other edges of your elbows, pressing your elbows against your hands to broaden your shoulders. Now slowly begin to bend forward from your hips. As you come forward keep the neutral position of your spine until your back is in a tabletop position. In the last few degrees of the movement you can allow the back to round softly as you release over the front leg and rest the forehead or nose on the shin (Figure 62). Only in this final variation should you round your back slightly. Work

---

SAFE TRANSITIONS

As you transition into and out of forward bending postures, be careful to support your back by drawing the soft frontal body up into your spine. Imagine your entire digestive tract, from mouth to anus, forming a line parallel to your spine. Keep your digestive tract in contact with your spine as you go down and as you come up. Thrusting your throat and belly forward as you go down, and hanging the organs off your spine as you come up, places undue strain on your back, requiring your back muscles to work overtime. Always use your whole body in concert when you transition into and out of forward bends.

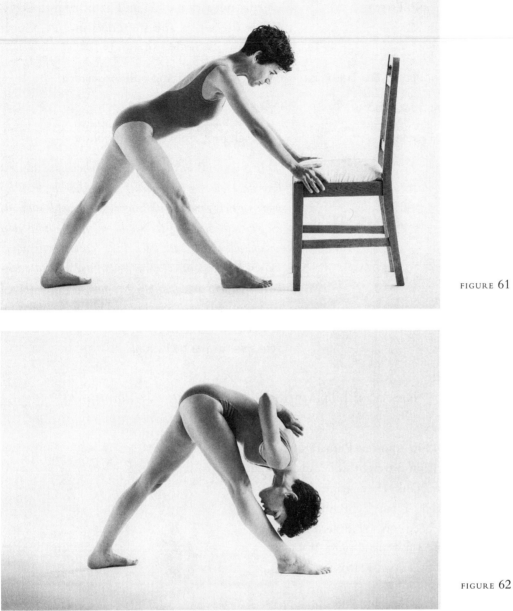

FIGURE 61

FIGURE 62

at whatever stage of the forward bend allows you to maintain the integrity of your spine for about ten breaths. Press down through your feet to come up, drawing your front body into your back body to prevent strain on your spine as you ascend.

Variation

If you can tip forward only 45 degrees, rest the top of your head against a wall (with a cushion between your head and the wall). Using your head as a sixth limb, you can press through the top of the head and lengthen through your spine. Supporting the head makes this variation easier on your back muscles, and allows you to feel the clear line of force from the crown of the head to the back heel.

BENEFITS AND EFFECTS	Deeply releases the hip and hamstring muscles. Keeps the wrists and shoulders mobile. Cools and calms the body and mind.
WHO SHOULDN'T DO THIS POSE	Those with hamstring pulls or sciatica.
PRENATAL SUGGESTIONS	⊕
HAVING TROUBLE?	My back foot comes off the ground.
TRY ...	*This is normal in the beginning when you are less flexible. However, all students can anchor the back leg more securely through utilizing greater organic support. As you are standing facing the front leg, draw your abdominal organs back toward the front of your spine. When the contents of your belly have shifted backward, you will automatically feel your weight anchored in your back leg. Sustain the parallel connection between the entire length of your digestive tract and your spine as you tip forward.*

Revolved Triangle Pose (*Parivrtta Trikonasana*)

Here's How

Stand in adjusted Preparatory Stance II on the right side (as you did for Flank Pose, page 106). Revolved Triangle Pose is a hybrid between Triangle, Flank Pose, and a full spinal twist. If you haven't practiced Flank Pose, go back now and do this posture as a preparation.

As you stand facing your right leg, inhale and extend your left arm over your head. Reach up and back until you feel a strong opening from your hand all the way through your belly and groin on that side (Figure 63). Slowly revolve your entire torso to the right as you bend forward from your hips. Sustain the connection between your sitting bones and your heels, being especially careful that you do not allow the

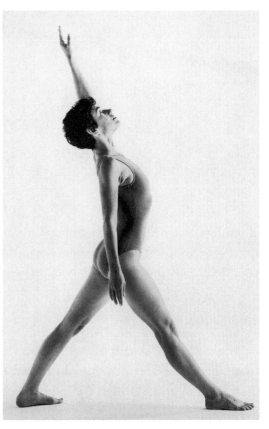

FIGURE 63

right hip to veer off the line of the right heel. In the beginning it will be difficult to bring the hand all the way to the floor, so adjust by raising the hand on a block placed on the *inside* of your right foot (Figure 64).

Imagine yourself as a starfish again, with the core of your body opening so the limbs can extend freely. Start by establishing a free, rhythmic breath, allowing your belly to open. Then work to feel the connection from your belly to your head and tail so that your spine elongates with each exhalation. Once you have established this core opening, your arms and legs will naturally extend freely outward. If you have difficulty feeling your torso turn, bring your top arm down and place your hand on your belly. On an exhalation use your hand to encourage the rotation through your core. Then, move your hand up to the middle of your torso, encouraging the center to rotate, and so on, until you are using your hand to coax your heart and lungs to come into the twist as well. Complete the movement in the last few breaths by turning your head to look at the outstretched arm (Figure 65). As you stay, inhale and anchor your legs, exhale, elongate, and twist your spine.

Variation

Beginners: If your back heel does not reach the floor, try wedging the heel in the corner of a room so your heel has full contact with a supporting surface. If you find the twist difficult or lose your balance easily, stand flush to a wall with your right foot forward. As you turn you will be facing the wall. You can use your right hand against the wall to guide your spine farther into the twist while checking your balance.

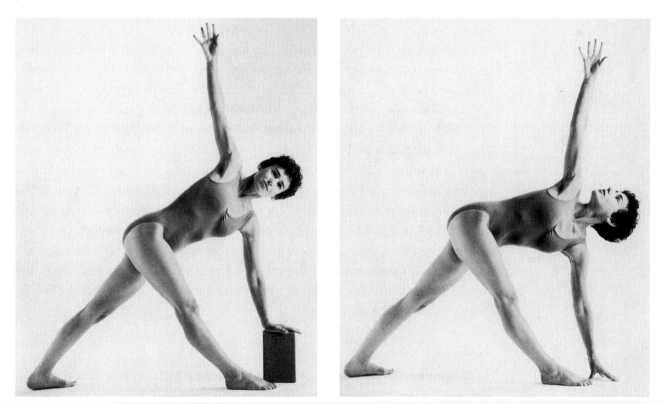

FIGURE 64   FIGURE 65

BENEFITS AND EFFECTS	Provides deep opening for the hip and hamstring muscles. Full spinal twist releases tension in the back. Stimulates the kidneys.
WHO SHOULDN'T DO THIS POSE	Those with acute back pain.
PRENATAL SUGGESTIONS	
HAVING TROUBLE?	I don't seem to be able to twist very far.
TRY . . .	*You are probably rounding your back and holding your breath. Lengthen the space from the base of your sternum to your pubic bone. This will free the diaphragm and allow your back to elongate so you can twist farther.*

Half-Moon Pose (*Ardha Chandrasana*)

Here's How

Stand in the Preparatory Stance II and take Triangle Pose (page 98) to the right. This is the precursor posture to Half-Moon Pose. Slowly bend your right knee, reaching your hand onto a block placed on the floor beyond your right foot or, if possible, with your fingers on the floor (Figure 66). As your weight shifts over your supporting leg, let your back leg drag slightly along the floor. On a deep exhalation come up onto your supporting leg, pressing down through your foot to anchor your weight into the earth. From this strong foundation let your belly blossom outward, extending all six limbs freely into space (Figure 67).

This posture is an extraordinary example of the principle of navel radiation. If your center is contracted and you are holding your breath, your limbs will be disconnected from your trunk. To establish the support from your center, bring your top arm down and use your hand to encourage the abdomen to open. You can put your back against a wall if you feel unsteady in your balance. Wait until you feel your core malleable and your breathing free before you attempt to extend your upper arm again. Finding the core support in this posture can take time, as it is all too easy to hold your breath in your attempt to master the balance. Be patient and be willing to experiment to find out what you need to do to both balance and breathe! This skill will stand you in good stead in difficult *asanas* to come.

To come out of the pose, slowly bend your supporting leg, and lower your back foot to the floor, returning to the original Triangle position. As your back foot touches, keep your torso parallel to the ground while you straighten both legs. Now practice on the other side.

Variation

Beginners: Many beginners find that their front hip cramps in this posture. If this is so for you, it's likely that you turned your front foot inward as you began to come up. This has caused your hip to rotate inward and our old friends the sitting

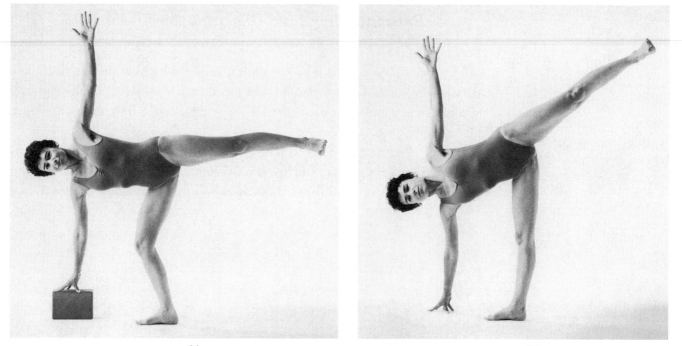

FIGURE 66   FIGURE 67

bones to be thrust well behind your heels. Practice the posture with your back to the wall while you make these corrections: As you come up, plant your foot downward, correcting any tendency for it to shift. Concentrate on tracking your knee clearly over the foot as you bend the knee, keeping it in a narrow corridor of movement throughout your ascent and descent. Once you are balanced over the leg, resist the tendency to rotate the opposite hip back so strongly that your hip muscles contract. Last, imagine your pelvis as riding buoyant and light on the legs so there is space between the pelvis and the femur.

BENEFITS AND EFFECTS	Refines balance. Tones the lateral muscles of the spine and legs. Increases circulation of blood around the liver, spleen, and stomach. Excellent for those recovering from hepatitis and mononucleosis, when done with a wall behind the back for support.
WHO SHOULDN'T DO THIS POSE	Those with hamstring tears should be cautious.
PRENATAL SUGGESTIONS	(Not for those with varicosities.)
HAVING TROUBLE?	I can't seem to balance.
TRY . . .	*Practice with your body facing a wall and rest your fingertips lightly against the wall. Check that the length of your body is parallel to the wall and not cantilevered toward or away from the wall.*

Expanded-Leg Pose (*Prasaritta Padottanasana*)

Here's How

This forward bend is easier on the spine and on the backs of the legs than those postures where your feet are placed closer together. It is ideal for people who have tight hamstrings and tight backs but feel vulnerable when they attempt to open either of these areas.

Begin in Preparatory Stance II with your feet *very* wide apart. The wider apart your feet, the easier the *asana* will be on your hamstrings. With your hands on your hips, slowly begin to bend forward on an exhalation. As you revolve from your

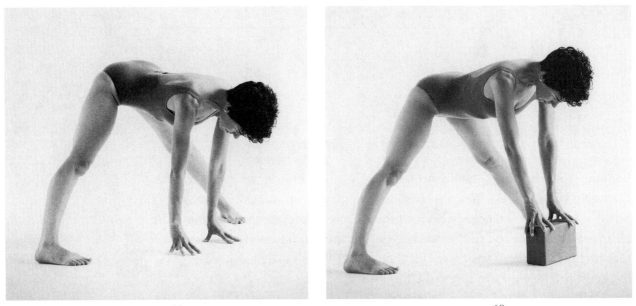

FIGURE 68   FIGURE 69

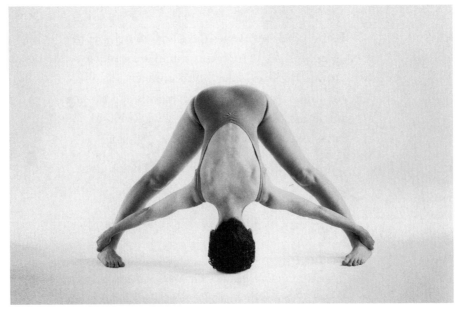

FIGURE 70

hips, maintain the long line of the spine from head to tail. Place your fingertips on the floor underneath your shoulders (Figure 68). If in coming forward, your back has rounded, raise your hands up onto a block (Figure 69). It is more important to maintain the elongation of the spine and the open position of your diaphragm than it is to touch your hands to the floor.

Keeping your weight centered on your feet, slowly release farther forward, moving entirely from the hip joints. As you are able to deepen the bend, bring your hands back underneath you so your fingertips are now in line with your toes. Slowly bend your elbows, releasing the shoulders away from the ears as you bring your head to the floor. For the final variation, clasp the ankles, and allow your lower back softly to round as you bring your head to the floor to complete the *asana* (Figure 70).

Variation

For a more intense variation, bring the hands behind your back in prayer position *Namaste,* just as you did for Flank Pose (page 106). This variation is suitable only for those who can comfortably rest their head on the floor.

BENEFITS AND EFFECTS	Releases the hamstrings. Gentle inversion—brings fresh blood to the head and rests the heart. Cools and calms the mind.
WHO SHOULDN'T DO THIS POSE	Those with disc herniations should be cautious. Those with glaucoma or detached retina should not lower the head below the level of the heart.
PRENATAL SUGGESTIONS	
HAVING TROUBLE?	My feet seem to slip apart.
TRY . . .	*Turn your feet farther inward, and narrow the width of your stance.*

Forward Stretch (*Uttanasana*)

Here's How

Stand in Mountain Pose with your feet hips-width apart. Slowly tip forward from your hips, generously bending your knees as you do so (Figure 71). Allow your entire spine to hang forward over your legs, gently opening the backs of your legs. Stay here for about ten breaths, focusing on releasing the weight of your head, neck, and arms so that your torso elongates. To come up, rotate your torso around the hips, bringing the arms out to the sides and over your head on an inhalation. As you exhale, lower your arms and return to Mountain Pose.

If you found the previous movement easy, try coming into the movement with straight legs, gradually deepening the bend from your hips on each exhalation. Imagine the sitting bones and the tail lifting upward as your pelvis revolves deeply

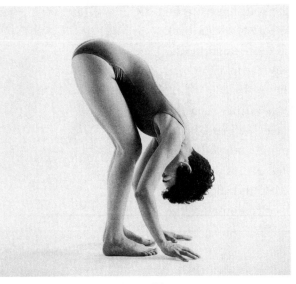

FIGURE 71

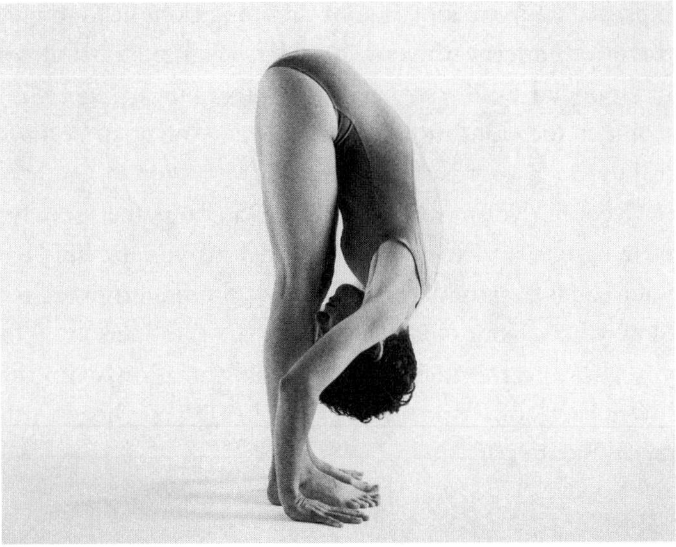

FIGURE 72

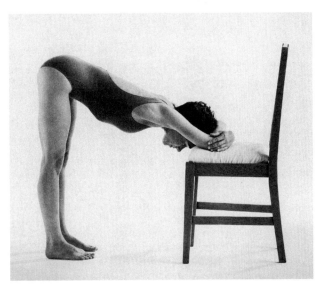

FIGURE 73

around your femurs. As you stay, focus on broadening the muscles along the backs of your legs, initiating this action by widening through the soles of your feet. Then broaden through the backs of the calves and through the plumpest part of your thighs. When you stretch only from the origin to the insertion of the hamstring muscles (from sitting bones to knees), the stretch will feel "sharp" and intense. As you learn to broaden the muscles from side to side, the stretch will feel diffused and thick.

Gradually progress from touching your fingertips to the floor, to lowering the palms onto the floor in front of your feet. As your legs open even more, you'll be able to bring the hands back to either side of the feet and release the head to touch the fronts of the shins (Figure 72).

Variation

Supported Forward Stretch (*Salamba Uttanasana*) This variation is wonderful when you feel those late-afternoon energy slumps and that all-too-common accumulation of tension in the upper back. Place a chair against a wall with the seat facing you. Bend forward from a standing position so that your elbows are crossed above your head with your forehead resting on your arms or the seat of the chair (Figure 73). If the chair is not cushioned, place a folded towel under your forehead for comfort. You can do this variation with bent or straight legs, depending on your hamstring flexibility. With each exhalation soften and release the muscles throughout the back, shoulders, and neck. Stay as long as you like, and when you wish to come up, bend your knees and walk your feet slightly closer to your head before pivoting up.

BENEFITS AND EFFECTS	Provides deep opening for the hamstrings, promoting freedom of the pelvis and back. Gentle inversion stimulates blood flow to the brain. Cools and calms the nervous system.
WHO SHOULDN'T DO THIS POSE	Those with herniated discs should be cautious.
PRENATAL SUGGESTIONS	⊕. (Trimesters II and III can do the supported variation with the feet wide apart to accommodate the belly.)
HAVING TROUBLE?	My hamstrings are so tight I can't relax!
TRY ...	*Try the Spinal Roll variation sitting on a chair (page 95) or the Half-Dog Pose (page 97).*

Standing Twist

Here's How

This is a very simple, safe twist that you can do frequently throughout the day to release your back. Because you are standing, your hamstrings place relatively little pull on the pelvis, allowing your spine to lengthen upward without restriction. Therefore this twist (unlike seated variations) places relatively little strain on your intervertebral discs and can usually be practiced even by those with disc problems. Let your own experience, however, be your guide. If twisting irritates your back, do not persist.

Stand with your right shoulder touching a wall. Place a chair with its back against the wall. Now bring your right foot up onto the chair. Press down through your supporting leg, elongating up through the crown of your head. Imagine your spine like a spiral staircase. As you inhale elongate the spine upward, stepping up the staircase, and as you exhale begin to spiral through the spine, turning toward the wall. With your right arm outstretched on the wall, use your left hand against the outside of the right knee to guide your spine into the twist (Figure 74).

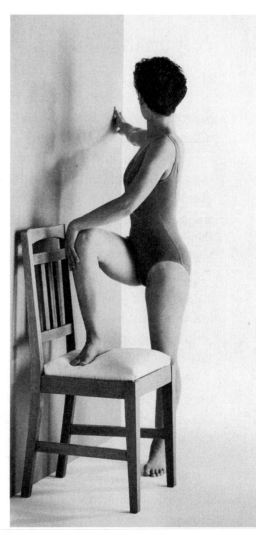

FIGURE 74

Be careful not to overrotate your head and neck, focusing instead on spiraling through your trunk.

If your back is very stiff, do this twist briefly (for ten to fifteen seconds) and repeat several times on each side. Otherwise, practice for one minute on each side.

Variation

Instead of standing, sit sideways on a chair and place your hands on the back of the chair. Guide your spine into the twist on each exhalation. This is a good variation for those who spend long hours doing sedentary work.

BENEFITS AND EFFECTS	Releases deeply held tension in the spine. Helps to reduce thoracic kyphosis (exaggerated curvature of the upper back). Eliminates fatigue and stiffness from the back.
WHO SHOULDN'T DO THIS POSE	☺
PRENATAL SUGGESTIONS	🕎

Downward-Facing Dog (*Adho Mukha Svanasana*)

Here's How

This is an *asana* that no yoga student ever outgrows. It's the garlic of yoga—a panacea for whatever ails you, which combines the benefits of an inversion, arm balance, forward bend, and restorative pose all rolled into one.

Begin by coming onto all fours with your hands resting slightly in front of your shoulders on the floor. Spread your fingers wide apart to distribute the weight evenly across your hands. To warm the shoulders and hips, turn your feet under and push off from your feet until your chest is over your hands (Figure 75a), and then push back from your hands until your buttocks are pressed down toward your heels (Figure 75b). Slowly rock back and forth to loosen and open the limbs.

On your next exhalation press away from the floor and lift the knees up, reaching back with your sitting bones and tail. Your arms and torso will be in one long line from your hands through to your tail (Figure 76). With each outgoing breath yield the weight of your arms to the ground as you simultaneously lift your pelvis up and back off your spine.

As you deepen in the posture rotate the shoulders outward. This releases the neck and upper thoracic spine and allows the force coming up through the arms to be communicated to the torso (Figure 77). If you rotate your shoulders inward, this restricts the neck and upper thoracic spine and prevents the flow of force from your arms through to your shoulder blades (Figure 78).

As you stay in the posture gradually release your heels down toward the floor. To come out of the pose, slowly bend your knees and relax into Child's Pose (page 193) with your arms by your sides.

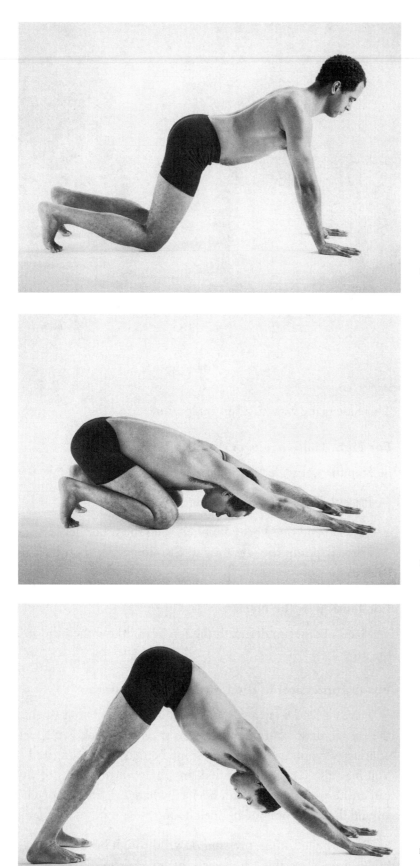

FIGURE 75A

FIGURE 75B

FIGURE 76

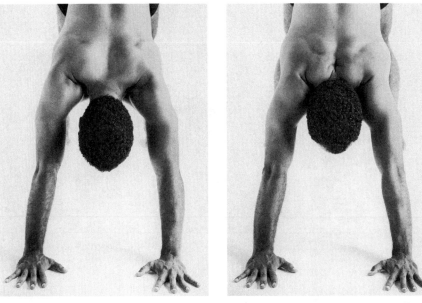

77. Correct   78. Incorrect

Variations

There are many ways to adapt this posture.

For Tight Hamstrings or Achilles Tendons

～ Step the feet wider apart and/or bend the knees slightly.

～ Place the heels up against a wall.

～ Slowly bend one knee while releasing the other heel toward the floor. Alternately pump the legs four to five times, and then try bringing both heels to the floor together.

For Tension in the Neck

～ Place a bolster underneath the forehead. Allow the head to release into the support.

For Compression in the Lower Back or Fatigue

～ Have a friend wrap a yoga tie around the tops of your thighs and pull on the ends to draw your thighs back. As they draw back you'll feel the weight coming off your arms and your spine being gently elongated (Figure 79). You may also feel an intensified stretch down the backs of your legs. You can create your own traction device by hanging from a yoga belt wrapped around the doorknobs of an open door.

～ Bend the left knee, pressing down through both hands to anchor the body. From this stable base, reach the tail over to the left. This will stretch and release the entire right side of your body (Figure 80).

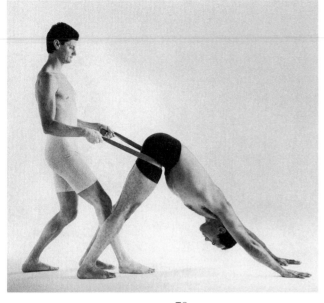

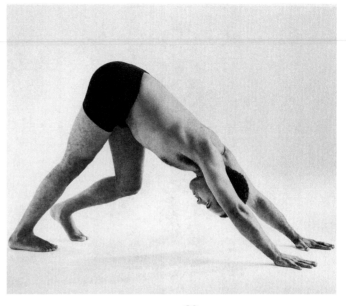

FIGURE 79   FIGURE 80

BENEFITS AND EFFECTS	Strengthens the wrists, arms, and shoulders. Elongates and releases tension throughout the entire spinal column. Stretches the backs of the legs and opens the hips.
WHO SHOULDN'T DO THIS POSE	Those with injuries to the wrists and carpal tunnel syndrome. Those with high blood pressure, glaucoma, or detached retina. Those with recent disc injuries should start with Half-Dog Pose.
PRENATAL SUGGESTIONS	
HAVING TROUBLE?	I feel pressure at the base of my wrists.
TRY . . .	*You are collapsing your weight into the base of the wrist. Place a rolled-up towel underneath the base of your forearms so that it is lightly touching the underside of your forearms just above your wrists. As you practice the pose lift your forearms upward as if to avoid touching the towel. This upward action will shift the weight forward to the front of the palm and throughout the fingers, taking the pressure off your wrist joint.*

Upward-Facing Dog (*Urdhva Mukha Svanasana*)

Here's How

Upward-Facing Dog is usually entered from either Downward-Facing Dog (page 116) or from Four-Limb Stick Pose (page 122). In this posture the spine is

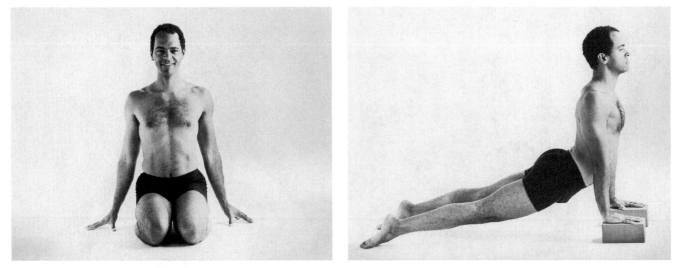

FIGURE 81   FIGURE 82

carried like a sway bridge between the pillarlike support of the arms and legs. If your upper back, groin, and shoulders are tight, there will be a tendency to seesaw on your lower back, extending too much from the lumbar while the other segments of the spine remain unengaged. Because this is such a common problem when attempting this posture, we will learn Upward Dog in stages. Do not progress to the next variation until you can practice the current one with a feeling of lightness and ease in your lower back. No pain is your gain!

Let's first try the movement without the stress of carrying your body weight through your arms and legs. Kneel with your hands on either side of your hips. Turn your hands to face slightly outward so you can rotate your shoulders without restriction. Draw the base of your shoulder blades downward, anchoring your arms strongly into the earth. This downward movement will encourage your spine to ascend. As the spine elongates upward, draw forward from your breastbone as if your chest were the masthead of a ship coming through your arms. In this first variation let your chin stay level as your chest lifts upward (Figure 81). This will teach you to open the stiffer upper back rather than simply extending from your neck. When your breastbone is vertical or beyond, then and only then slowly extend your head back into an arc, releasing the throat forward.

In the next stage you'll practice the posture with blocks underneath your hands. Raising your hands decreases the acuteness of the angle in the lower back, making this a safer option for beginners. Start from Downward-Facing Dog (page 116) with your hands raised on blocks. Slowly shift your weight forward and through your arms, drawing your chest over the support of your arms (Figure 82). If your chest is behind the support of your arms, when you press down through your arms, you will be pushing back into your lumbar spine (Figure 83). Turn onto the tops of your feet so that your knees and hips are off the floor. See yourself as the human starfish again, now turning itself inside out with head, tail, arms, and legs extending away from the opening navel. Keep your head level until you can

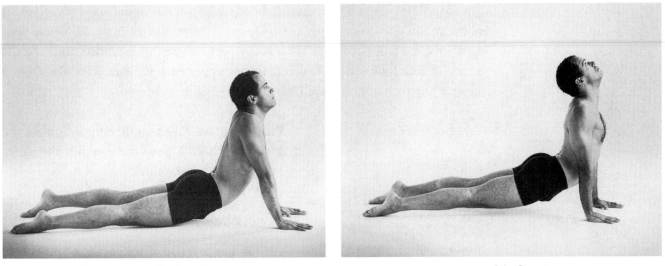

FIGURE 83. *Incorrect*   FIGURE 84. *Correct*

practice the posture with a fully elongated back, breastbone vertical. When you have accomplished this, you can briefly extend the head back to complete the *asana*. Stay for five deep breaths, focusing on elongating from the crown of the head through a smooth curve in your back, all the way out through your legs to the tips of your toes. Then transition back into Downward-Facing Dog, taking a few moments to release the back in the opposite direction. When you can practice this stage on the blocks without discomfort in your lower back, bring your hands onto the floor for the classic posture (Figure 84).

Variations

For Those with Stiff or Sore Wrists

∼ Practice the posture with the hands on the outer edges of the seat of a chair. Curl your fingers under the chair with the thumbs on top. This will put your wrists in a more neutral position. Or use a wrist wedge under the base of your palms (see page 28).

For Those with Weak Arms and Legs

∼ Practice the posture with your knees touching the floor.
∼ Work on building arm strength by practicing Downward-Facing Dog and Four-Limb Stick Pose.

For Those with Compression and Pain in the Lower Back

If lifting your hands onto a block and actively reaching through your legs does not diminish this sensation, it's likely that you are hinging on the mobile segments of your back (lumbar and neck) without ever addressing the tightness in your upper back. Rather than try to solve this problem in Upward-Facing Dog, take a few weeks (or months) to practice deep lunges that open the front of your groin (see pages 104–6), and passive back-bending movements (see pages 182–84) that allow you to open your upper back. Opening the segments above and below your lumber spine will encourage their active participation in extension and take the stress off your lower back. As you feel your upper back loosening, it's likely you'll be able to return to practicing Upward-Facing Dog without pain.

BENEFITS AND EFFECTS	Provides powerful strengthening action for the arms and chest. Opens and expands the chest. Heats and builds stamina.
WHO SHOULDN'T DO THIS POSE	Those with carpal tunnel syndrome. Those with spondylolisthesis or spondylolysis.
PRENATAL SUGGESTIONS	Do not practice if you feel a pulling sensation in the rectus muscle (the central abdominal muscle running from the base of your sternum to your pubic bone). This muscle should not be compromised during pregnancy by overstretching in back bending, because it may separate or tear, making postpartum recovery of the abdominal muscles difficult.
HAVING TROUBLE?	See variations.

Four-Limb Stick Pose (*Chaturanga Dandasana*)

Here's How

Unlike many yoga postures where the focus is on increasing flexibility, this *asana* is all about keeping everything in one piece. The hands and feet touch the ground while the body is suspended above the ground in one unit or "stick," as in the calisthenic push-up. Just like Upward-Facing Dog, it teaches you to use your limbs to support your spine. It is usually practiced as a transition posture between Downward- and Upward-Facing Dog as a part of the Sun Salutation.

Begin in Downward-Facing Dog (page 116), focusing on connecting your head and tail through your central core. In this first variation you will lower the knees to touch the floor. As your knees touch the floor, release your buttocks back to touch your heels. Your chest will now be closer to the floor than your abdomen. Maintaining this relationship, thrust forward from your feet to bring the chest forward and over the support of your arms (Figure 85). The key is to bring your chest down toward the floor *before* the abdomen. The other essential trick is to bend your elbows the moment you begin to shift your weight forward. If you bring your chest and head all the way forward over straight arms, your arms must now carry your full body weight as you lower yourself to the floor. Attempting to lower your torso from this position takes considerable arm strength and invariably leads to col-

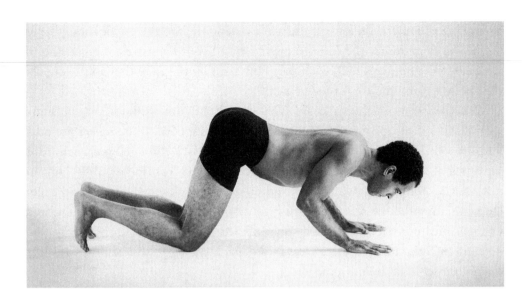

FIGURE 85

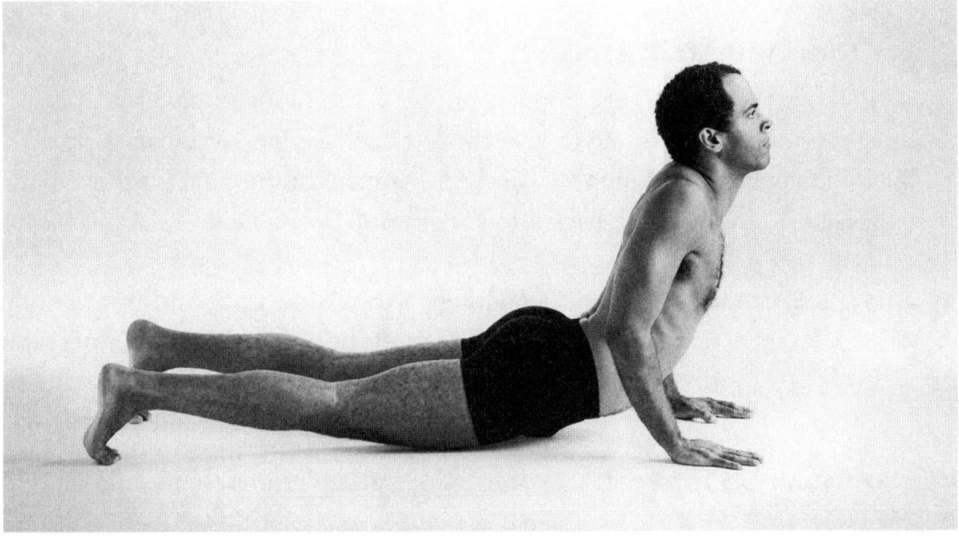

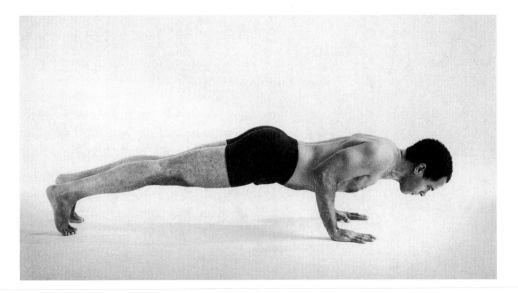

FIGURE 86. *Incorrect*

FIGURE 87

lapsing the abdomen and lower back while extending into the upper back (Figure 86). If you synchronize the forward movement of your chest with the bending of your elbows, your arms will be already fully bent by the time they must support your body weight, and that's much easier!

This first stage, with your knees still resting lightly on the floor, may be sufficient challenge for those still building upper-body strength. To complete the posture, lift your knees off the floor and reach strongly back through your heels. Your torso will now be suspended over your active arms and legs (Figure 87). Maintain this position for one or two breaths and then push back into Downward-Facing Dog, initiating the transition by lifting your abdomen up toward your spine and strongly pushing back through your arms. As you become stronger you can descend into the posture from Downward-Facing Dog Pose, keeping your legs straight throughout the movement.

Variation

For Those with Weak Arms

∽ Practice the "plank" position by shifting your chest forward over your straight arms without trying to lower yourself to the floor. Maintain a clear line from your head through to your heels. Sustain this position for three to five breaths, and then push back into Downward-Facing Dog.

BENEFITS AND EFFECTS	Strengthens the wrists, arms, and upper body while toning the abdominal muscles. Increases overall stamina and endurance. Brings a sense of vigor and lightness to the body and mind.
WHO SHOULDN'T DO THIS POSE	People with carpal tunnel syndrome should avoid this *asana*.
PRENATAL SUGGESTIONS	(Only if you were practicing the posture with ease *before* you became pregnant.)
HAVING TROUBLE?	Try as I may, I cannot lower my body without collapsing into a heap.
TRY . . .	*It's likely that you are allowing your organs to "hang" from your spine instead of staying parallel with your back. Practice the inquiries in the "Back-Bending" section (see pages 176–79) and then attempt the posture again, keeping your focus on sustaining the connection between the inner "tube" of your digestive tract and the outer rod of your spine.*

Sun Salutation
(*Suryanamaskar*)

Here's How

The Sun Salutation is practiced as one continuous flowing motion, alternating expanding and condensing movements in a symbolic enactment of our dual connection to the life-giving sun and earth. When you first begin your practice, you may feel like spending a minute or more in each position to warm the body. As you do successive cycles you can gradually reduce the time you spend in each position until you are flowing from one full movement to the next.

There are many different versions of *Suryanamaskar* and traditionally the cycle is practiced with a predetermined breathing pattern. In the variations here, I've made suggestions about when to inhale or exhale in coordination with your movements, but these are meant only as suggestions and not as rigid rules. Watch how your breath pattern spontaneously changes in response to the speed with which you practice the cycle and how the breath matches the shape of the movements—rising and expanding or descending and folding.

You can begin your practice with this cycle to warm your body and stimulate your circulation. You can also alternate Sun Salutations with standing postures, or insert the standing postures *inside* the cycle itself to link the postures in a flowing sequence.

Beginner's Variation
(This variation requires less upper-body strength
and is especially good for those with weak backs.)

1. Mountain Pose (Figure 88): Stand in Mountain Pose. As you exhale, bend your knees slightly, anchoring your weight into the earth. As you inhale, uncoil your back fully by pressing down through your legs. With your palms curled inward graze the backs of the fingers together as you bring your hands in front of your face (Figure 89), opening the palms outward as the arms curve upward over the head. Follow your arms with your gaze (Figure 90).

2. Forward Stretch (Figure 91): Exhale and bring your hands into a prayer position, down past your face and chest to the floor. Keep your knees bent and let your spine hang between your thighs. Use the exhalation like an anchor, feeling the weight of it drop down through the spine and out through your head. In more challenging variations of the Sun Salutation the forward bend will be one of the only resting positions in the cycle. Learn to let go completely and relax your head and neck to take full advantage of this restful position.

3. Lunge (Figure 92): On an inhalation, step the right leg back behind you, allowing the knee to rest lightly on the floor. The leg that you step back will be the leg that you later bring forward to complete the cycle. With each cycle, lunge back on a different leg.

4. Downward-Facing Dog (Figure 93): As you exhale, step the left leg back and press back through your arms as you reach up and out through your hips. If your legs are very tight, step your feet farther apart. Stay on the balls of the feet with the heels lifted to make the position easier on your lower back and hamstrings. Stay here as you take a deep inhalation.

5. Extended Child's Pose. As you exhale touch your knees to the floor, and reach your buttocks back toward your heels. Press your palms firmly into the ground to open the shoulders (Figure 94).

6. Transition to Upward-Facing Dog Pose (Figure 95): On your next inhalation slide your chest down and through your arms. Be careful to use your arms to support your back rather than allowing your back to sag as you descend.

7. Upward-Facing Dog Variation (Figure 96): Replace your arms so you are now resting on your forearms like a sphinx. Inhale as your chest comes forward and through your arms. Press your elbows back toward your feet to assist the forward action of your spine. Turn your feet under and reach back through your legs, working to create a smooth curve through your back up to the crown of your head. Do not bring the head back in this variation, but work instead to draw the chest and sternum into a vertical position.

Return to

8. Downward-Facing Dog (Figure 97): On an exhalation, replace the hands under the shoulders and press back into Downward-Facing Dog.

9. Lunge (Figure 98): On an inhalation bring the right leg forward.

10. Forward Stretch (Figure 99): On an exhalation.

11. Mountain Pose (Figure 90, then 88): On an inhalation sweep the arms up and out to the sides and over your head. As you exhale return them to your sides. You have now completed one cycle of *Suryanamaskar.*

Sun Salutation (The Classic Variation)

1. Mountain Pose (Figure 100): On inhalation.

2. Forward Stretch (Figure 101): On an exhalation bring your hands into a prayer position down past your face and chest to the floor. In this variation the legs remain straight, intensifying the stretch through the back of the body.

BEGINNER'S SUN SALUTATION

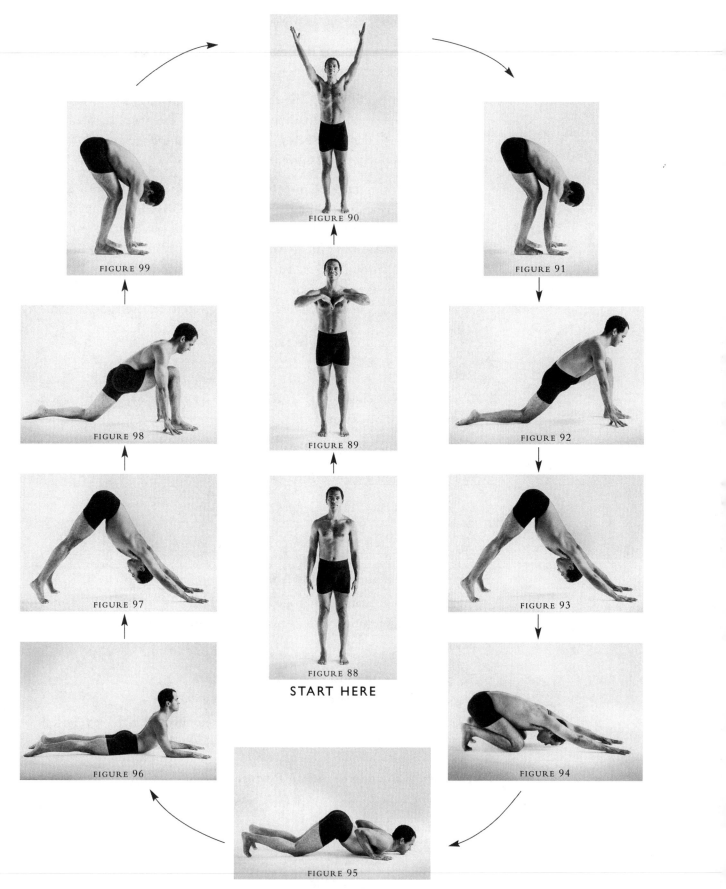

FIGURE 90

FIGURE 99

FIGURE 91

FIGURE 89

FIGURE 98

FIGURE 92

FIGURE 97

FIGURE 88

START HERE

FIGURE 93

FIGURE 96

FIGURE 94

FIGURE 95

3. Lunge (Figure 102): On an inhalation lunge the right leg back.

4. Downward-Facing Dog (Figure 103): On an exhalation. Now begin to descend the heels toward the floor.

5. Four-Limb Stick Pose (Figure 104): On an exhalation push back through your feet as you dive the chest through the arms, drawing the elbows in close to the ribs. Keep your heels reaching back to create a strong counterforce to the forward movement of your chest.

6. Upward-Facing Dog (Figure 105): On a deep inhalation press down through your hands, straightening the elbows and drawing the chest forward and up through the arms. As you make the transition turn onto the tops of the feet one at a time. Reach back through your toes as you press strongly down through your arms to create a platform for the spine to ascend. Keep the eyes level with the horizon until you can establish a vertical chest, and then, and only then, allow the head to release back to complete the posture.

Return to

7. Downward-Facing Dog (Figure 106): On an exhalation push back and up into Downward-Facing Dog.

8. Lunge (Figure 107): On an inhalation lunge the right leg forward.

9. Forward Stretch (Figure 108): On an exhalation.

10. Mountain Pose (Figure 100): On an inhalation.

Variations

To Strengthen and Tone the Abdomen and Legs:

~ Practice Horseman's Pose (page 96) at the beginning of the cycle. After a breath or two, transition into Forward Stretch by releasing the arms down to the floor.

To open the hips and release the lower back (especially as a preparation for arm balances):

~ Add a deep squat at the end of the cycle before you straighten your legs for Forward Stretch.

To create a flowing Standing Posture/Sun Salutation Sequence:

~ Insert any standing posture into the cycle after your lunge. The cycle will go as follows:

1. Mountain Pose (see Figure 100, page 129).

2. Forward Stretch (see Figure 101, page 129).

Classic Sun Salutation

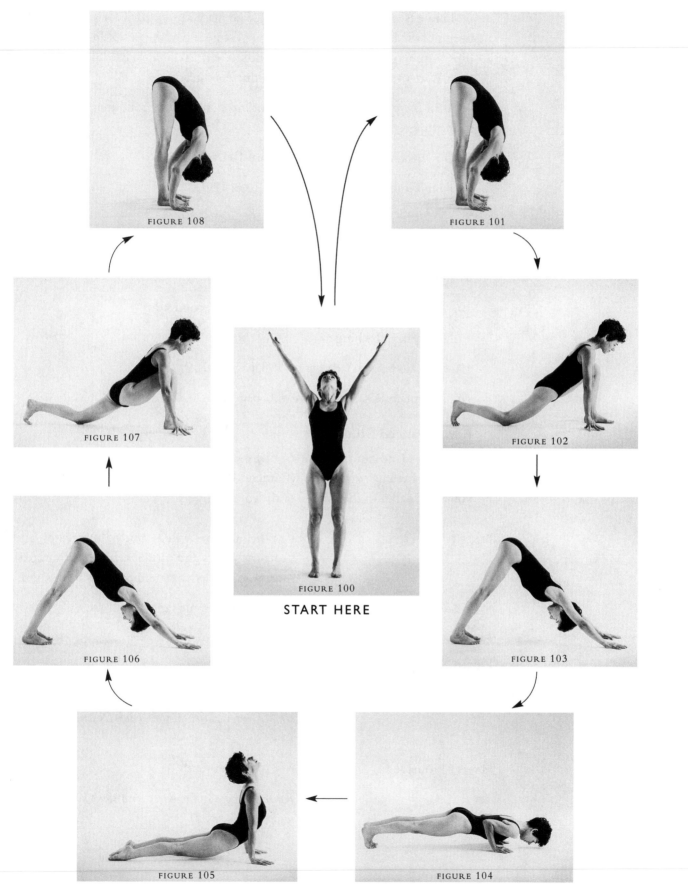

FIGURE 108

FIGURE 101

FIGURE 107

FIGURE 100

START HERE

FIGURE 102

FIGURE 106

FIGURE 103

FIGURE 105

FIGURE 104

3. Lunge (see Figure 102, page 129). The leg you step back for your lunge becomes the back leg of your standing posture. Pivot the pelvis around your hips to practice the pose of your choice (e.g., Triangle Pose, Side-Angle Pose, Warrior Pose). Stay for three to thirteen breaths.

4. Turn the pelvis back over the front hip, bending the front knee to return to the lunge.

5. Downward-Facing Dog (see Figure 103, page 129).

6. Four-Limb Stick (see Figure 104, page 129).

7. Upward-Facing Dog (see Figure 105, page 129).

8. Downward-Facing Dog (see Figure 106, page 129).

9. Lunge (see Figure 107, page 129).

10. Now take your standing posture on the second side.

11. Return to the lunge.

12. Forward Stretch (see Figure 108, page 129).

13. Mountain Pose (see Figure 100, page 129).

For Advanced Students:

∾ Add a Handstand (page 216) or Elbow Stand (page 218), at the end of the cycle before returning to Mountain Pose. Practice this variation only if you can balance in the middle of the room.

BENEFITS AND EFFECTS	Conditions the whole body. Lubricates and heats the joints and muscles. Improves circulation. Reduces lethargy and combats depression.
WHO SHOULDN'T DO THIS POSE	Those with chronic fatigue.
PRENATAL SUGGESTIONS	(symbol)
HAVING TROUBLE?	My back hurts in Upward-Facing Dog.
TRY . . .	*Leave out the Upward-Facing Dog altogether and simply lunge forward after your Downward-Facing Dog.*
HAVING TROUBLE?	My wrists get sore!
TRY . . .	*Raise the base of the wrist on a slant board or wrist wedge (see page 28)*

IV
The Sitting Postures—
Forward Bends and Twists

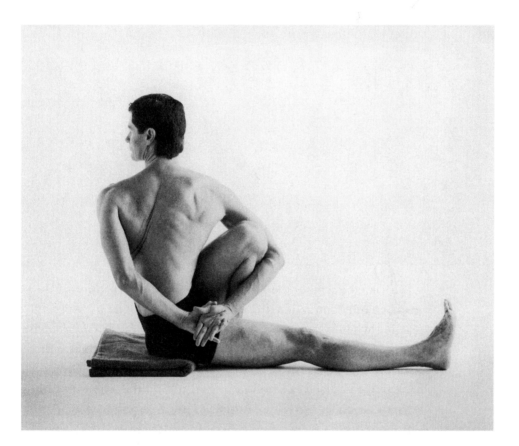

INTRODUCTION

*L*ike the symbol the spiral, which begins its expansion at the point of maximum contraction, the spiritual journey is one in which the destination is reached when we return to the self. Or as the *Tao Te Ching* advises: "Going on means going far, going far means returning." These postures represent just such a return to the self. As we bend forward or twist our bodies we curve our awareness back toward ourselves, looking inward to find the stillness of our center. As we learn to surrender and release into that return, we can recuperate from the outward actions of our busy everyday lives, taking solace in self-reflection. This movement inward is like the coiling action of the spring, and is the necessary precursor to our uncoiling into our next project, activity, or growth spurt. Without it, we can become like elastic that has been stretched too far: unable to return to its original length, it loses its ability to hold things together.

Many people begin practicing hatha yoga with the belief that one elusive day, when they have touched their toes or achieved a particularly difficult posture, they will be doing "good" or "real" yoga. In truth it matters little how far you can bend forward or how far you can twist, for wherever the point of resistance lies is the place where you have the greatest opportunity to learn and to change. This opportunity exists whether you have the flexibility of an ironing board or the mobility of a gymnast. If you can meet yourself just where you are rather than always looking beyond yourself to where you'd like to be, this attitude of steadfastness and compassion will bring the fruits of yoga to you.

On a physical level the forward bends release all the muscles along the back of the body—the notorious hamstrings and the spinal muscles. The action of bending forward is restful for the heart and cooling and calming for the body and mind. Twisting the body opens the spine at its deepest level, releasing locked-in tension. Whenever you've done a lot of bending forward or backward, twisting, even briefly, brings the spine back into a neutral state. Through the squeezing-and-soaking action that comes when the internal organs are alternately compressed and released, toxins and excess heat are expelled, and fresh nutrition is brought to these vital powerhouses.

KEY MOVING PRINCIPLES FOR THE FORWARD BENDS

1. BREATHE
Let the Breath Move You

2. YIELD
Yield to the Earth: Weight and Levity

4. CENTER
Maintain the Integrity of the Spine: The Central Axis

ESSENTIAL SKILLS

Sitting Well: Stick Pose (*Dandasana*)

The Pelvis: Finding Your Base of Support

All of the sitting postures are born out of one posture—the Stick Pose (*Dandasana*). To sit well you must learn to sit on the center of your sitting bones. The *ischial tuberosities* lie underneath the flesh of your buttocks, and when you sit on them (rather than the spine itself), the pelvis becomes a very effective base of support. As you yield your weight through the sitting bones, the rebounding force will move up into your pelvis and back, creating an upright posture (Figure 110).

Your hamstring muscles attach to the base of the pelvis, and if they are very tight, they will draw the pelvis under, causing you to sit on the back of your sitting bones and sacrum. This inevitably causes your spine to round, putting pressure on the delicate discs and making it impossible to sit comfortably (Figure 111).

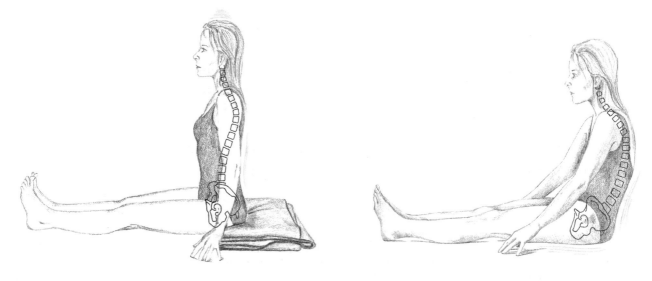

110. *Correct*   111. *Incorrect*

There are a number of ways you can improve your sitting, even if your hamstrings are tight. The first is to raise your pelvis with a folded blanket. This changes the carrying angle of your trunk, making it easier to find that "sweet spot." Additionally you can bend your knees slightly, which releases the grip of the hamstrings on the pelvis, allowing your pelvis to rotate forward into an upright position (Figure 112). You can use these two strategies in any sitting posture to make the task of sitting both easier and more pleasurable.

∾ INQUIRY ∾

Centering the Weight Through the Pelvis

Start by sitting on your yoga mat with your legs extended in front of you. Bring one hand onto your lower back and feel whether the lumbar vertebrae are curving outward or whether they are slightly indented (see Figure 14, page 42, for an understanding of spinal curves). If your back is rounding, you are most definitely sitting on the back of your sitting bones. Now place a folded blanket (or two) underneath your buttocks until you feel your back come upright. Take your hands under your buttocks and locate your sitting bones. They are hidden under pads of fat and muscle, but they are there! Draw the flesh of the buttocks back so that you can feel the contact of the sitting bones against the blanket, and then center your weight through them. If your pelvis is still rolling back, try bending your knees. This will allow you to rock forward with your pelvis to come into an upright position. Press your hands lightly into the floor on either side of your hips to assist

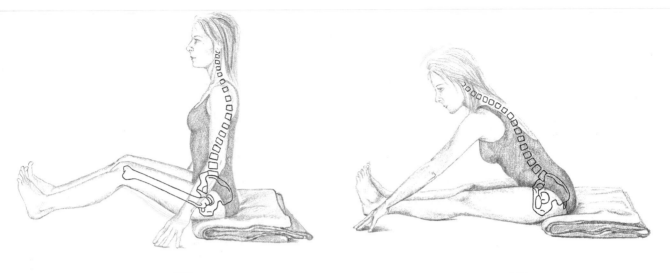

FIGURE 112   FIGURE 113

you. This centered position is the starting point for all the sitting and twisting postures.

Bending Forward: Moving from Your Hips

When you bend forward, the action should be initiated by the movement of your pelvis revolving around your thighbones (Figure 113). When the pelvis is able to rotate around the femurs, the lumbar curve will remain in a neutral position throughout most of the action, reversing only at the very end of the forward bend. While it is normal for your lumbar curve to reverse when your torso hinges close to your legs (or your legs hinge in toward your chest), it is not normal for this reversal to happen at the beginning of your forward bend. If your hamstrings are very tight, they may limit this action, causing the pelvis to remain fixed around the hips. This will cause your lumbar spine to reverse its curves at the *beginning* of the movement, which places extreme pressure on the intervertebral discs.

Spinal Reach of the Head and Tail

The other part of this equation is that when you bend forward, it's essential to maintain the length of your spine, reaching out through the head and down and back through your tailbone. While it is tempting to come forward by rounding the back and drawing your head down in a snail-like fashion, this way of working is injurious to your spine and never truly addresses the areas of the body that are restricted. Elongation means space, and space means freedom in your joints, length in your muscles, and, most important, room to breathe. By maintaining the conditions that support free breathing, you allow the breath to do the work of opening your body.

∼ INQUIRY ∼

Bending Forward with Ease

Sitting on a chair, place your hands on your pelvis with your fingers touching the hipbones in the front and thumbs wrapped around the back of the pelvis. Position your feet slightly wider than your hips on the floor in front of you. Place your weight through your sitting bones and reach through the top of the head. Imagine your torso as the hand of a clock and the pelvis as the central dial. As you tip forward, maintain the length through your spine, letting the fulcrum of the action come from the pelvis revolving around the femurs. Check with your hands that your pelvis is the central mover with the spine going along for the ride, rather than simply hinging from your back. Tip forward as far as you can, maintaining the length in your back. In the beginning you may not be able to go very far before your back rounds. Stop just before you feel this happen. Notice how the sensation of stretching is coming from your hips and your legs rather than your spine. To come up, reach down and back with your tail, anchoring your weight into your sitting bones.

Now fix the position of your pelvis and bend forward from your spine (do not attempt this if you already have a back injury). Notice that your only choice as you come forward in this way is to round your back. Observe how quickly it becomes difficult to breathe in this compressed position and how all the sensation is centered in your back. Return to the neutral position and try coming forward again from your hips. Compare the difference between these two ways of moving.

Descending the Femurs

Part of what allows you to bend freely forward from your hip sockets is the actual space between your femur and your pelvis. Regardless of whether you are bringing the torso down toward the legs as in Head-to-Knee Pose (page 143) or whether you are bringing the legs in toward the chest as in Reclining Big-Toe Pose (page 138), the action is exactly the same. Whenever you bend forward, the tops of your thighbones should *descend* away from your shoulders. In Figure 114 you can see how the femur is moving down and back out of the pelvis, even as the leg is drawn in toward the chest. This action creates enormous space in the joint and allows you to go much farther. In Figure 115 the person has drawn the femur up into the hip socket, causing compression in the hip. The leg now comes in toward your chest not because the hip is releasing but through the action of the whole pelvis being hiked up toward the shoulder on that side and through the side-bending action of the spine. If your hips and legs are tight, your body will always choose the easiest option—going around the restriction of the hips by bending through the lumbar spine. You can encourage your femurs to descend in most postures by pressing your thumb strongly downward into the crease of the joint.

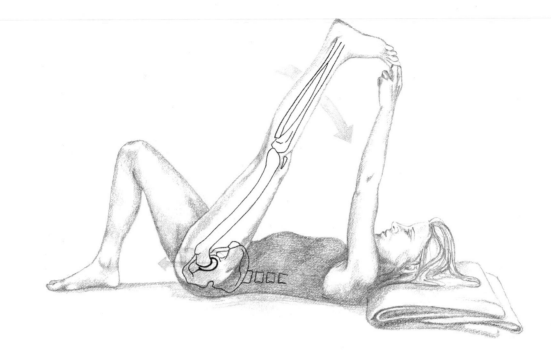

FIGURE 114. *Correct*

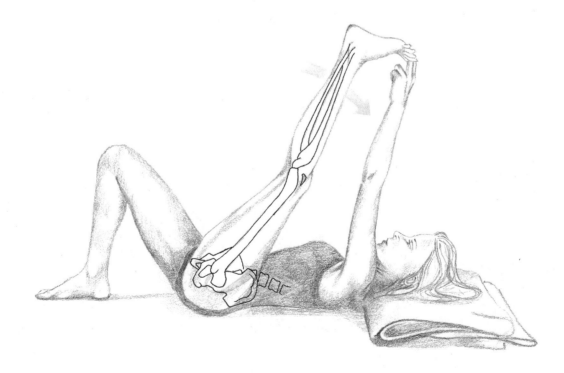

FIGURE 115. *Incorrect*

~ INQUIRY ~

Descending the Femurs

To learn this skill, practice the first forward bend in the following series.

THE FORWARD BENDS

*(Unless otherwise suggested, you'll want to have a few
blankets and a yoga tie for all postures in this chapter.)*

Reclining Big-Toe Pose (*Supta Padangusthasana*)

You'll Need

A wall

Here's How

Reclining Big-Toe Pose is one of the mainstays of hatha yoga practice. Because you are reclining, the spine is in a relatively neutral position, allowing you to lengthen your hamstrings without challenging the back. The following variations are meant to be done as a progressive series.

Variation A

Lie on your back with your knees bent and your feet facing a wall. If your head and neck are arching back, place a folded towel or blanket under your neck to the edge of your shoulders until your forehead is slightly higher than your chin. Now draw your right knee into your chest, clasping the shin (or the back of your thigh) with both hands. Feel the rhythm of your breath expanding and condensing your abdomen. This expanding and condensing action is actually moving the pelvis, spine, and leg very slightly. As you breathe out, feel how the movement inferred by the breath invites the leg to come closer to your chest (Figure 116) and how as you breathe in the leg moves away from your chest. Connect with this guiding rhythm, gently rocking the leg in and out. This is an excellent movement if you have a very stiff or painful back, and can be practiced while still in bed in the morning to loosen and release your hips and spine.

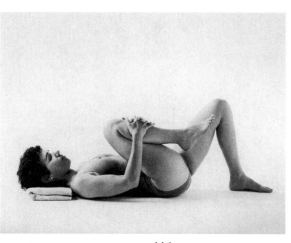

FIGURE 116

Variation B

The next step is to slowly straighten your right leg, placing a tie around the sole of your foot. As you straighten the leg check that the femur is descending away from your shoulders. Bring your right thumb into the crease of the hip and encourage the femur to descend. This will free the hip. Now, with each successive exhalation, invite the leg to come toward you (Figure 117). If you are unable to bring the leg to at least 90 degrees or more, the hip will tend to move up in the socket. If this is the case for you, bend your leg a little while still drawing it toward the chest. If your leg is at a right angle or more, you are ready for the next variation.

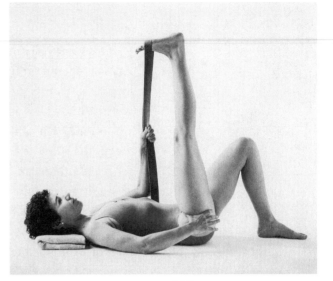

FIGURE 117

Variation C

Now slowly extend your left leg along the floor. As the sole of your left foot makes contact with the wall, press firmly into the wall. This contact with the wall will allow you to move force through your leg into your torso, lengthening your entire body as well as giving you a strong opening through the front of the left groin and thigh. Continue to encourage the right femur to descend, using your right hand if necessary. If your leg is at a right angle or more, you may be ready to take hold of the big toe. Only do this if you can keep your shoulders relaxed on the floor as you hold the foot (Figure 118). Stay here for at least a minute, inviting your leg to come closer to your chest on each exhalation.

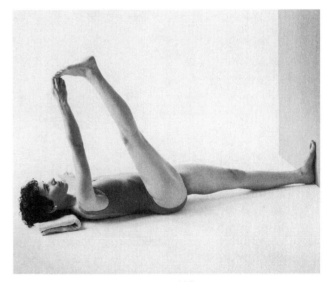

FIGURE 118

Variation D

Now, keeping your navel facing directly upward, turn your right leg out and open it to the side. If you are unable to keep your pelvis from tipping to the side, try bending your left knee again and opening that leg out to the side so the two legs are like the pages of an open book. Extend your left arm in line with your shoulder along the floor to give yourself even greater stability. Eventually you'll be able to bring the right leg up and out to the side while holding the big toe. Until then, use the extra help of the tie (Figure 119). After a minute bring the leg back in to a neutral position.

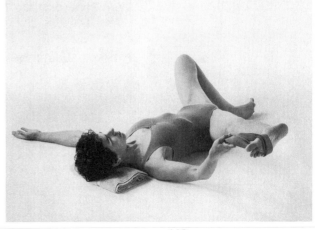

FIGURE 119

Variation E

This final variation gives the hip a deep internal stretch and creates a strong diagonal opening across the trunk to the opposite shoulder. On an exhalation take your tie in your right hand (or hold the big toe . . .) and slowly cross your left leg over the body, allowing yourself to roll onto your right side (Figure 120). If this is too intense, you can bend the right knee. As you extend through your left leg, check that the femur is still descending in the socket and your hip has not hiked up toward your shoulder. Reach back with the opposite arm, creating a strong diagonal twist through your torso. To release the shoulders and upper back toward the floor, adjust your shoulder blades by "walking" them away from your spine so your weight rests as much as possible on the inner border of your scapula. Stay for a minute, breathing low and slow into your belly. Now take the series on the second side.

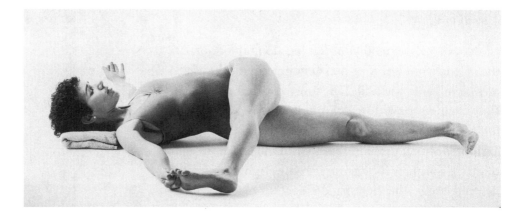

FIGURE 120

BENEFITS AND EFFECTS	Lengthens and releases the hamstrings and lower back. Provides a full-body twist, stimulating the spinal column and the organs of elimination.
WHO SHOULDN'T DO THIS POSE	Those with disc herniations or sciatica should be cautious.
PRENATAL SUGGESTIONS	After Trimester I lying flat on the back is not advised (page 85). You can do the same movements in a standing position by raising one leg up onto a chair or low ledge and slowly hinging forward over your leg.
HAVING TROUBLE?	The backs of my knees hurt.
TRY . . .	*Try bending your knee, and when you do straighten your leg, imagine the plumpest part of your leg muscles broadening with the action.*

SIMPLE SITTING

Sitting with ease and with a light, erect carriage is one of the lost arts of modern civilization. The ability to align the body with the supporting surface of the earth and with the field of gravity allows us to remain in a relatively still position for long periods of time with ease and dignity. This is an essential skill whether you choose to practice it at your computer or while sitting in meditation.

There are many ways to sit, apart from the classic Lotus Pose. Sitting with legs crossed twists the spine slightly to one side, so whichever sitting position you choose to work with, remember to alternate the cross of your legs during your practice so that your hips and spine develop evenly.

Tailor's Pose (*Sukhasana*)

For most Westerners accustomed to sitting on chairs, sitting on the floor with legs crossed is a challenge. The key to comfort is to raise your pelvis with folded blankets or a meditation cushion until your knees are slightly lower than your hips. You'll know you have the correct propping when your thighs release out of your pelvis and your abdomen relaxes (Figure 121).

Sage Pose (*Siddhasana*)

In this position you draw one foot in toward your perineum, with the other foot resting on the ankle and lower calf of the other leg. The top foot will lie comfortably in the fold between the calf and thigh of the other leg (Figure 122). Many people find Sage Pose easier than the Tailor's Pose. Experiment with both to see which suits you.

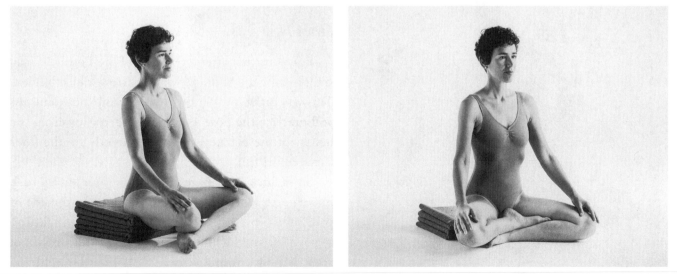

FIGURE 121 FIGURE 122

BENEFITS AND EFFECTS — Opens the hips and strengthens the back. Provides a stable position for meditation practices. Calms and settles the mind.

WHO SHOULDN'T DO THIS POSE — Sitting puts a great deal of weight through the discs. Those with compressive injuries or conditions of the lower back and hips should practice reclining leg stretches, standing postures, and standing forward bends until these are comfortable before working on sitting.

PRENATAL SUGGESTIONS — (Use a wall behind you for extra support if you feel tired.)

HAVING TROUBLE? — I get tension in my upper back when I sit for more than a few minutes.

TRY . . . — *Focus on yielding the weight of your sitting bones into the floor to anchor your posture and create a natural rebound through your back, rather than trying to "lift" your back into an upright position. You can also sit with your back against a wall until your back muscles become stronger.*

Cow-Face Pose (*Gomukasana*)

Cow-Face Pose is an excellent way to improve your sitting because it gives a deep opening to the hips as well as providing a great release to the shoulders. It is best done a number of times on each side, and is especially nice as a starting movement for your practice.

Here's How

For your first attempt at Cow-Face Pose you may want to raise the buttocks with a narrow folded blanket. This will make it easier on your hip and knee joints. As you practice the pose a second time, try lowering the height of the blankets or sitting directly on the floor between the feet.

Sit in Stick Pose (page 133). Draw your left leg back underneath you with your left foot on the outside of your right hip. Now bring your right knee over the top of your left knee, with your right foot on the outside of your left hip. Your buttocks will now be centered between the two feet. Place your hands on top of the

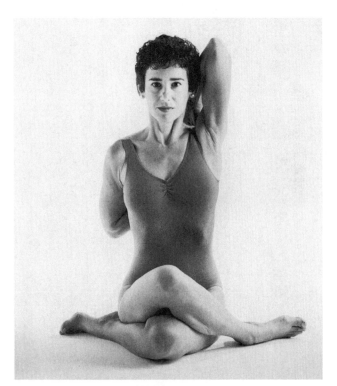

FIGURE 123

right knee and press down gently to further open the hips. Breathe! This can be an intense pose the first time around as you experience the strong sensation of the hips opening. Now extend your right arm to the side, bending the elbow to bring your arm behind your back. You can use your other hand to help move the hand in toward the spine and up toward the head. Then extend your left arm over your head, bending the elbow and clasping the left and right hands together (Figure 123). If you can't reach your hands, drop a yoga tie from your top hand down to the bottom one. Clasping the tie, extend the two ends of the tie away from each other. Stay here for at least one minute, breathing into both your hips and shoulders. Then do the second side. If you have time, repeat each side at least once more.

BENEFITS AND EFFECTS	Reduces stiffness in the shoulders and hips. Opens the chest and reduces congestion in the lungs.
WHO SHOULDN'T DO THIS POSE	☺
PRENATAL SUGGESTIONS	(Raise the buttocks higher as your pregnancy progresses, so that your abdomen and groin are not pinched.)
HAVING TROUBLE?	I feel pain inside my shoulder joints.
TRY . . .	*When the shoulders are very tight, I recommend using a rubber latex "Dynaband" instead of a yoga tie. These bands have more "give" than the ties and can be bought through a physical therapist; they are sometimes available at aerobic centers. If the pain persists, see your health professional.*

Head-to-Knee Pose (*Janu Sirsasana*)

This pose is not so aptly named, as the true destination is to bring the head to the shin rather than the knee. Keep this in mind as you come forward.

You'll Need

Possibly a bolster or folding chair

Here's How

Sit in Stick Pose (page 133), raising your buttocks if necessary to bring your weight squarely on your sitting bones. Now draw your right knee back and out to the side, bringing your right foot to the inside of your left thigh. Depending on your hip flexibility, your two legs will form a 90- to 130-degree angle. If your right knee has come up off the floor, place a rolled-up sock or towel underneath it for

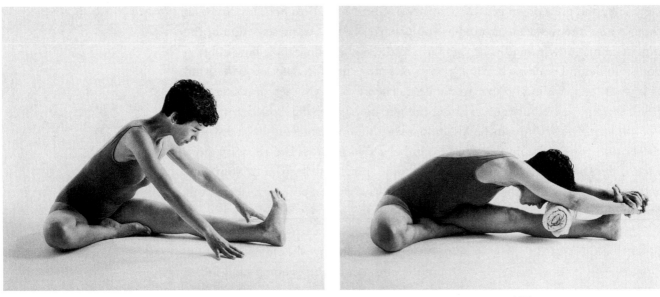

FIGURE 124   FIGURE 125

support. Take a breath in, and as you exhale, slowly begin to tip forward from your hips. If your pelvis doesn't budge, bend your left knee. Reach through the top of your head and maintain the length through your spine, resting your hands lightly on the floor on either side of your left leg to support you (Figure 124). In this beginning variation of Head-to-Knee Pose, your back muscles are working strongly against gravity. Stay for up to a minute, keeping your breastbone lifted so you will have room to breathe. If this is as far as you can go comfortably, complete the posture by resting your forehead against the edge of a chair (page 241) or on a bolster placed across the shin of the extended leg.

If you are able to go farther forward while maintaining the length through your abdomen and spine, reach your hands around the ball of your left foot and clasp the back of your right wrist with your left hand. Your palms will be facing away from you. Allow your breath to oscillate your spine so that it is lifted and lowered with each breath. Follow these undulations, encouraging the spine to stretch out over the left leg, eventually bringing your forehead to rest on your shin. If you can't come down this far, place a folded towel or cushion on your shin to support your forehead so you can enjoy the restfulness of this final position (Figure 125).

BENEFITS AND EFFECTS	Opens the hips and spine. Tones and stimulates the abdominal organs and the sex glands. Cools the body and calms the mind.
WHO SHOULDN'T DO THIS POSE	Those with disc problems should be cautious.
PRENATAL SUGGESTIONS	As pregnancy progresses practice only the beginning of the posture with the spine upright.
HAVING TROUBLE?	My bent knee hurts.

TRY...

Torque on the knee is usually caused by restriction in the hips. Sit in Stick Pose (page 133). Flex your right foot and turn the leg out (like a ballet "first" position). Rest your heel against the inside of the left ankle. Your knee will be slightly bent. This position will allow you to open the hips without putting pressure on the knee as you bend forward in Head-to-Knee Pose.

Revolved Head-to-Knee Pose
(*Parivrtta Janu Sirsasana*)

Here's How

Variation Start in the preparatory position for Head-to-Knee Pose with your right leg bent and your left leg extended. Turn the torso in the direction of the right knee, opening the chest and broadening through the spine. On an inhalation, extend your right arm over your head and begin to reach toward the left foot, sliding your left hand out along the length of the left leg (Figure 126). Focus on expanding and elongating through your left lung, and with each exhalation let the right side of your body release over the leg. Imagine that as you breathe you are loosening the "soil" around the roots of your right arm, which lie deep in the trunk. Stay for about one minute, and then repeat the posture on the other side.

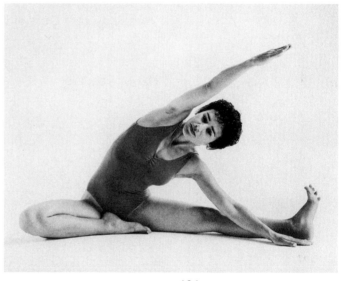

FIGURE 126

Final Position Start in the preparatory position for Head-to-Knee Pose with your right leg bent and the left leg extended. Again, turn the torso in the direction of the right knee, except this time slide your left arm forward along the floor in between your two legs until you are resting on the outside of the left shoulder. Carving an arc between the two legs, slowly stretch the left arm back along the floor toward the left leg, taking hold of the left heel by rotating the entire arm upward. Lengthen through the sides of your body as you extend the right arm over your head, now clasping the top of the left foot. As you release out over the leg, anchor the right hip toward the floor and reach back

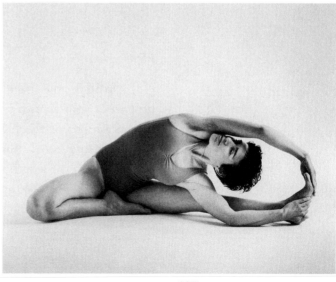

FIGURE 127

through your right knee. With each exhalation turn the entire torso to look up at the sky. Eventually you will be looking up underneath the right arm (Figure 127). Stay for up to a minute and then slowly release.

As you become more adept in Revolved Head-to-Knee Pose, you can secure your shoulder underneath the knee of the extended leg. To do this you bend your left knee, slide your left shoulder underneath it, and then slowly extend all the limbs outward as you straighten your leg. Anchoring the shoulder will allow you to rotate the spine even more effectively. In this variation it can be helpful to place a small pillow underneath the head so you can relax your neck as you hold the posture for a greater duration.

BENEFITS AND EFFECTS	Stretches all the lateral muscles of the body. Releases the intercostal muscles—improves breathing. Invigorates the entire body.
WHO SHOULDN'T DO THIS POSE	Those with disc problems should be cautious.
PRENATAL SUGGESTIONS	
HAVING TROUBLE?	I feel a strong pull along the side of my shoulder and body.
TRY ...	*Place a chair to the side of your body next to your extended leg. Extend your underside arm onto the seat of the chair and reach the other arm over your head. Rotate the underside arm up toward the ceiling and focus on reaching up and out with both arms instead of trying to bend to the side.*

Wide-Spread-Angle Pose I and II
(*Upavistha Konasana* I and II)

Here's How

Sit in Stick Pose (page 133), finding your weight on your sitting bones. Use the support of your arms if necessary to bring your spine upright. Slowly spread the legs apart, opening the angle as far as you can without leaning back onto the backs of your sitting bones. Turn your knees to face up toward the ceiling and press down through the length of the legs to anchor your position (Figure 128a).

If you are able to sit upright with ease, you are ready to move into the forward bend. Hinging from your hips and maintaining a long line from your head to your tail, slowly bend forward. Use your hands for support. In the beginning you may be able to come forward only a few inches. No matter where you are in the continuum of the motion, keep your mind centered by anchoring your weight through your legs as you inhale and having the *intention* to come forward

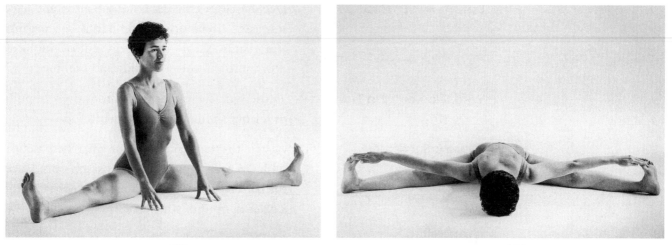

FIGURE 128A   FIGURE 128B

as you exhale. Eventually your chest will come all the way down to the floor (Figure 128b).

Wide-Spread-Angle Pose II

This variation is very much like Revolved Head-to-Knee Pose except here instead of turning the chest upward, you twist forward and down over one leg. Begin by turning from the waist and chest to look out over your right leg. Place your hands on either side of your leg and begin to hinge forward from your hips, reaching out forward through the head and back through your tailbone. As you extend over your leg, press down through the left leg, anchoring the thigh so the pelvis can move independently. Come down only as far as you can without losing the length through your spine. Eventually you will complete the posture by clasping the back of your left wrist with your right hand around the ball of your foot. Rest your head on the shin and stay for up to a minute, then repeat on the other side (Figure 129).

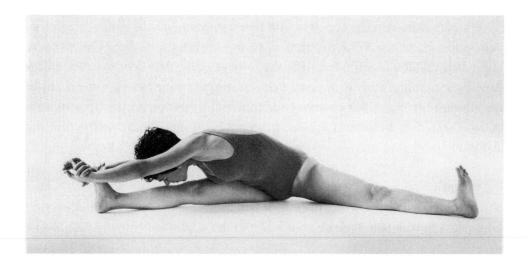

FIGURE 129

BENEFITS AND EFFECTS	Deeply releases the insides of the groin and legs. Increases circulation to the pelvis, sex organs, and glands. Moves the energy out of the head down into the core—cooling and calming.
WHO SHOULDN'T DO THIS POSE	Those with hamstring, adductor, or groin pulls or sciatica should be especially cautious.
PRENATAL SUGGESTIONS	⬙ In the later stages of pregnancy, practice with the back in the upright position only. Place the back against a wall, or support your hands on a chair in front of you.
HAVING TROUBLE?	I feel a strong pull on the backs of my knees.
TRY . . .	*Your hamstrings are making their presence known. Bend your knees and practice both the upright and forward bending positions, keeping the knees slightly bent, or place a rolled-up washcloth underneath both knees.*

Bound-Angle Pose (*Baddha Konasana*)

You'll Need

A block or a few telephone books

Here's How

Sit in Stick Pose (page 133). Bend your knees and, drawing your heels in toward your groin, bring the soles of your feet together. Maintaining the upright position of your back, clasp your feet (or ankles if you are tighter), and actively draw the knees out and down to the side (Figure 130). Stay for a few minutes in this position, gradually releasing the knees farther toward the floor.

Hinging from your hips, slowly fold forward. Maintain the distance between your pubic bone and your sternum so your breathing stays free. Once you've come halfway down you'll find that the lumbar curve naturally reverses. Allow your back to round slightly as you reach out through your head (Figure 131). In the advanced stages of this posture your chin will be resting on the floor in front of your feet. Stay here for a minute or more, breathing low and slow into the abdomen.

Variation: To access a different opening of the hip, raise your feet onto a block. Support yourself with your hands behind you on the floor, and draw your groin close to your feet. Release your knees to the side.

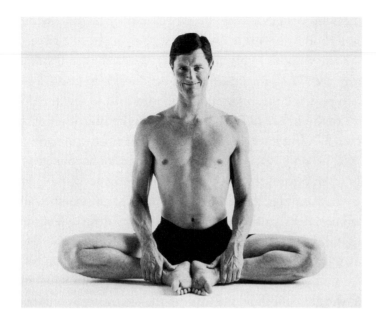

FIGURE 130

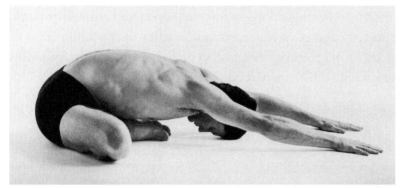

FIGURE 131

BENEFITS AND EFFECTS	Releases the hips, groin, and lower back. Strongly increases circulation to all the organs of the pelvis. Powerful preventive and restorative posture for symptoms related to premenstrual, menstrual, menopausal, and prostate disorders.
WHO SHOULDN'T DO THIS POSE	Those with sprained ankles.
PRENATAL SUGGESTIONS	This is a powerful prenatal pose and can be practiced every day unless there is incompetence of the cervix or pelvic floor.

Lotus Posture Preparations

Sitting comfortably in Lotus Pose depends on one thing—the openness of your hips. Unlike our Indian friends, however, we did not grow up sitting on the floor, and consequently our hips have developed in adaptation to life in chairs.

Additionally, the hip is an extremely deep ball-and-socket joint with some of the strongest muscles and ligaments in the body supporting it. The knee, on the other hand, is one of the weakest joints in the body. When the leg is straight the knee joint will not rotate. When the knee joint is bent as it is in Lotus, a slight rotation does come into play, and this rotation can be injurious to the knee. Similarly the ankles, relative to the hip, tend to be unstable. This combination of the stable hip and the structurally weak knee and ankle is the reason why so many people injure themselves trying to do Lotus Pose. If the opening is not encouraged from the hip but forcefully levered from the knee and ankle, the knees will be damaged long before you have a glimpse of the real McCoy. Any discomfort, especially sharp sensations in the knee, is a sign that you are working incorrectly and need to adjust your position. If this doesn't help, get assistance from an experienced teacher.

The following are preparatory movements for opening the hips for the Lotus Posture. These are best done after practicing standing postures, when the body is warm. Those who are tight should practice in the afternoon, when the body is naturally more flexible. Begin by practicing these preliminary movements for one minute, gradually staying as long as three minutes. And remember that changing your hip structure takes careful, persistent practice over a long period of time. If you work safely and correctly, eventually you *will* get into Lotus, and you will have healthy knees with which to celebrate your accomplishment.

Growing Your Lotus

- **The Swan** (Stretches the muscles of the external rotators of the bent leg, the illiopsoas muscles—the muscles responsible for lifting the thigh, as in walking—and the groin of the extended leg.)

Sit with the heel of your right foot in line with your pubic bone. Extend your left leg straight behind you with the kneecap facing downward. Draw your left hip toward the floor. Keep your chest lifted to take the weight of the pelvis off the femur (Figure 132). Sustain for one minute and then repeat on the other side. To intensify the opening, you can move your foot away from your thigh until the thigh and calf form a right angle in front of you.

- **Through-the-Hole Stretch** (Stretches the external rotators of the hip.)

Lie on your back with both knees bent. Turn your right leg out and place it across the top of your left thigh. Take your right arm through the gap of the right leg around the back of the left thigh or onto the left shin. Clasp hands. As you draw your left thigh toward you, turn the right hip out and move the right knee away from you to open the hip. This is the action of the legs in a good Lotus Pose. It's essential that you keep the right foot flexed so that you cannot see the sole of the foot (Figure 133). This deliberate stabilization of the ankle prevents you from levering the rotational action from either the ankle or knee and forces the opening to occur from the hip alone.

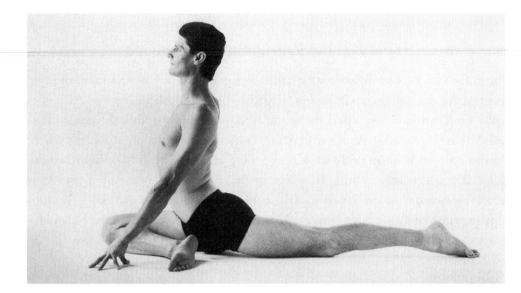

FIGURE 132

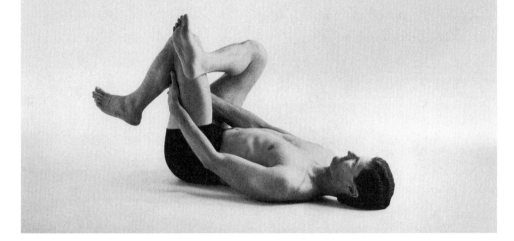

FIGURE 133

• **Cradle Stretch** (Stretches the lateral rotators and adductors.)

Sit in Stick Pose (page 133). Bend your right knee and turn your leg out. Raise your leg off the floor and place the sole of the foot in the crease of the left elbow and the thigh in the crease of the right elbow. Clasp hands. Gently move the hip back and forth, rotating the hip outward as you do so. To increase the intensity of the stretch, keep moving the right foot away from the floor until the leg forms a right angle (Figure 134). You are now in the starting position for Half-Lotus Forward Bend.

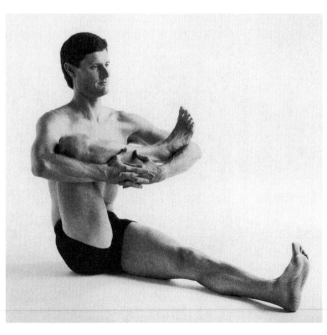

FIGURE 134

Half-Lotus Forward Bend
(*Ardha Baddha Padma Paschimottanasana*)

From the Cradle Stretch, place your ankle on top of your left thigh so that the heel is pressing into the lower abdomen. If you right knee is more than a few inches away from the floor, you will be better off wedging the foot against the ankle of the other foot (Figure 135). We have shown this variation from the other side for clarity. In this position you can safely work on opening up your hip without injuring your knee. If you were able to bring your foot up into the lower abdomen but your knee is still an inch or two off the floor, place a folded blanket under your knee. By supporting your knee in this way, you make it possible for the muscles of the hip gradu-

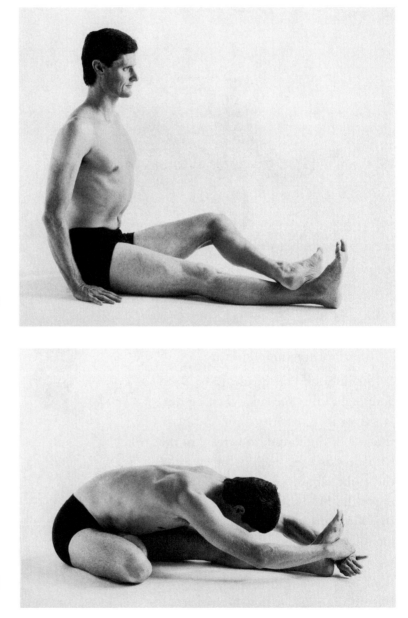

FIGURE 135

FIGURE 136

ally to let go. The movement of your knee toward the floor should be accomplished by a deep rotation in the hip socket, and not by twisting the ankle and torquing the knee. Go slowly, and do not move further into any of these variations if you experience pain in your knees—they are very unforgiving joints once injured.

Eventually you will be able to fold forward so that your forehead is resting on your shin and the heel of the lotus foot is giving the flexor points of the colon a deep massage (Figure 136).

These postures are also helpful warm-ups for Lotus Pose:

Wide-Spread-Angle Pose II (page 147)
Bound Angle with the feet elevated on a block (Variation, page 148)
Head-to-Knee Pose (page 143)
Cow-Face Pose (page 142)
Sage Pose II (page 164)

When bringing the foot onto the top of the thigh for Lotus Pose, hold your shin and ankle from *underneath the leg* so you are rotating the shin and thigh outward in the direction that your hip must turn. Never pull on the foot alone with the hands above the leg. Keep your ankle flexed, drawing the little toe of your foot back toward the outer knee to prevent the rotation from coming at the ankle or knee (Figure 137). Once your ankle is resting on your thigh, you may relax the foot. Supinating, or allowing the ankle to bend so that the sole of your foot faces up at you,

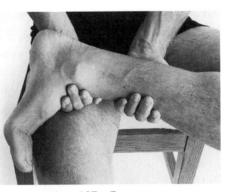

137. *Correct*

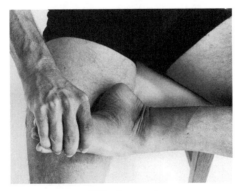

138. *Incorrect*

weakens the already vulnerable ankle and pulls on the ligaments and cartilage of the lateral knee, causing potential injury to these delicate structures (Figure 138).

Lotus Pose (*Padmasana*)

You'll Need

A towel

Here's How

This method of entering Lotus was taught to me by yoga master Dona Holleman. It is infinitely safer than the common strategy of tugging the second leg up into Lotus. If your Lotus knee was close to or touching the floor in Half-Lotus Forward Bend, you are probably ready to make an attempt at the Full Lotus. From Half-Lotus Forward Bend, with the right leg in Lotus, place your left ankle *underneath* your right knee. You are now in a Half-Lotus sitting position. Lean back until you are balanced on the back of your sitting bones, allowing your right leg to come off the floor. Now bring your hands underneath your left shin and point of the ankle joint. Slowly lift your left leg up off the floor, allowing the leg to be completely relaxed. Now instead of pulling this leg up and over the right leg, concentrate on releasing the *right* knee and thigh down toward the floor (Figure 139). Breath by breath, allow the right leg to rotate farther outward. When the right leg comes level or lower than the left, you will be able gently to slip the left leg over the top of the right. As you do so you can rest both legs back down onto the floor (Figure 140).

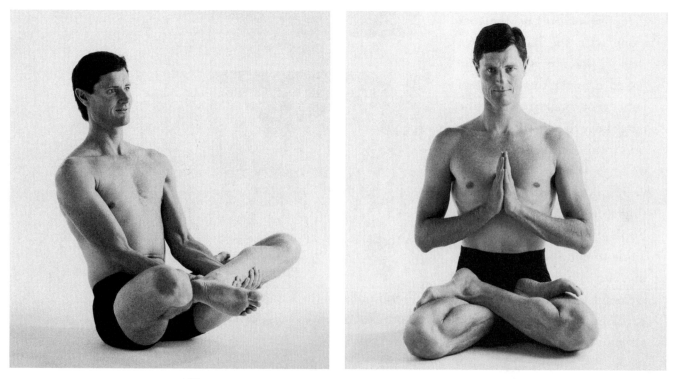

FIGURE 139   FIGURE 140

It's normal for the top knee in Lotus to be slightly off the floor. Place a rolled-up sock or towel under the knee if it is more than an inch away from the floor. Lotus is an asymmetrical pose, causing a slight rotation through your spine, so it's important to cross your legs both ways and to practice for equal lengths of time on both sides. If you cannot do the full Lotus on one side (as is commonly the case), it's important to work through all the preparatory movements as close to the final pose as you can.

BENEFITS AND EFFECTS	Opens and releases the hips. Provides a stable base for the spine in sitting meditation. Reduces swelling and water retention in the feet and lower legs.
WHO SHOULDN'T DO THIS POSE	Those with sprained ankles. People with current knee injuries should be particularly cautious.
PRENATAL SUGGESTIONS	
HAVING TROUBLE?	The top of my thigh where my ankle rests hurts!
TRY . . .	*When the foot is drawn up high enough on the thigh, it fits into a groove between two muscles. When there is insufficient flexibility to achieve this ideal position, the foot rests on the mound of the thigh muscles, making it uncomfortable for both ankle and thigh. This discomfort is rarely injurious and unfortunately is one of the stepping stones along the way into Lotus.*

West Stretch (*Paschimottanasana*)

Here's How

Traditionally the Sun Salutation was practiced at dawn, facing east to the rising sun. This made the front of the body the "east" side and the back the "west." In this posture the entire west side of the body receives a deep opening.

Begin in Stick Pose. Descend the weight of your femurs down into the ground as you allow your spine to float up. If you are a beginner, you may want to practice this pose with your knees bent until you can feel the pelvis rotating freely around your thighbones. Once the pelvis is able to move independently of the legs, straighten your legs and draw the trunk forward

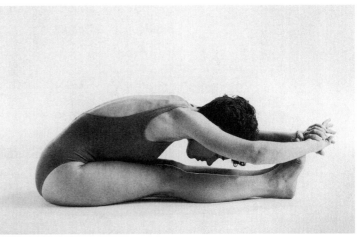

FIGURE 141

and out toward the feet. Use your hands on either side of the spine for support, going only as far as you can while keeping the abdomen long and released and your breathing free. This may be a few degrees off the vertical or the final position as shown (Figure 141). Wherever you are, allow your spine to oscillate with your breath, making sure you honor both the retractive phase of the breath that lifts you slightly out of the movement, and the releasing phase of the breath that allows you to deepen your position. Stay for one to three minutes.

BENEFITS AND EFFECTS	Releases all the muscles along the back of the body. Increases the circulation to the pelvic organs and sex glands. Draws the energy down, reducing anxiety and quieting the mind.
WHO SHOULDN'T DO THIS POSE	Those with disc injuries should be very cautious.
PRENATAL SUGGESTIONS	
HAVING TROUBLE?	I feel a strong pull on the backs of my knees.
TRY . . .	*Bend the knees or try working with a towel rolled underneath the knees. Concentrate on broadening the muscles through the thickest part of the thigh and calf instead of reaching through your heels.*

Boat Pose (*Navasana*)

Here's How

Although this is neither a forward bend nor a twist, the Boat Pose is a derivative of Stick Pose (page 133). It can be practiced as a part of almost any yoga sequence, but should be done only once your back has been strengthened through the standing postures, upright practice of sitting postures, and through the simple back bends such as Locust.

Long and Strong Abdominal Warm-up

Traditional sit-ups in which the abdomen bulges outward are good for neither the belly nor back. The focus in this preparatory movement is on lengthening the abdominal muscles as well as drawing them in toward the spine as you roll up. Start by lying on the floor with your knees bent. With your hands reaching toward your feet, imagine that you are holding an orange under each armpit (this will stabilize your shoulder blades). Slowly curl up one vertebra at a time, reaching out through the crown of your head as if you were curling around a large ball. Reach through your arms, grazing the sides of your thighs as you come up to a sitting position

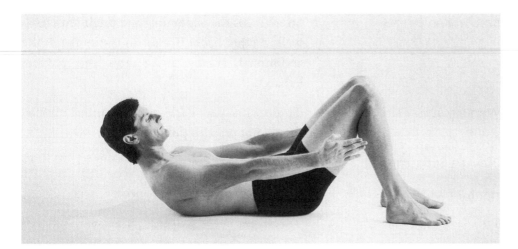

FIGURE 142

(Figure 142). If necessary, hold the sides of your legs. To come down, slowly reverse the movement.

Boat Pose

Once you are able to do the Long and Strong Abdominal preparations with ease for at least five repetitions, you are ready to try the Boat. Come up until you are balanced on your sitting bones with your hands clasping the back of the thighs. Maintaining your balance, slowly straighten your legs up and out in front of you. Let your gaze look slightly above your toes and, when you are confident, let go of your thighs and extend the arms strongly either side of each leg (Figure 143). Stay for at least three breaths, then rest your feet on the floor and slowly recline back to lying on the floor.

You can do repetitions of these two postures or practice holding the poses for longer periods of time.

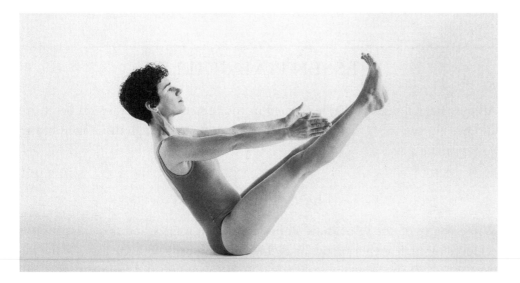

FIGURE 143

BENEFITS AND EFFECTS	Strengthens the abdominal and thigh muscles as well as the back. Tones and stimulates the abdominal organs. Invigorates and reduces lethargy.
WHO SHOULDN'T DO THIS POSE	Those with weak backs and abdominal muscles should not practice this posture.
PRENATAL SUGGESTIONS	Not Suitable.
HAVING TROUBLE?	I can't seem to find my balance.
TRY . . .	*This may be due to your body proportions—very long legs and a short trunk, for instance, will make this more precarious. Try practicing Boat Pose with your back 6 inches from a wall.*

THE TWISTS

Key Moving Principles for the Twists

1. BREATHE
Let the Breath Move You

2. YIELD
Yield to the Earth: Weight and Levity

4. CENTER
Maintain the Integrity of the Spine: The Central Axis

7. ENGAGE
Engage the Whole Body: Review the Organ System.

ESSENTIAL SKILLS

All the essential skills you have learned in your practice of the forward bends are also true for twists. Refresh your memory by glancing through those skills before you continue.

The Spiral Staircase

When you twist, the spine must elongate before it rotates, and this elongation is achieved through anchoring the body downward (usually with the legs and the sitting bones) while simultaneously releasing the spine up and following through

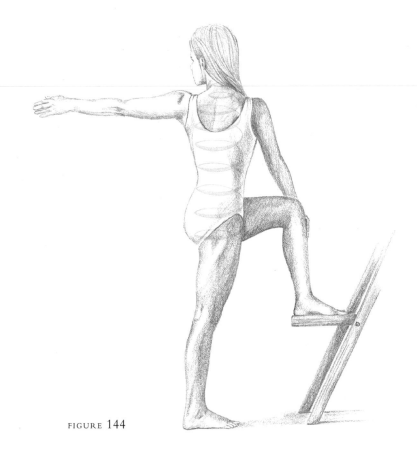

FIGURE 144

with a reach of the head. Imagine in every twist that there is a spiral staircase running through the central axis of your body. Just as you must step up as you ascend a spiral staircase, while you inhale, elongate your back upward, and while you exhale, turn into the movement. Pause in the space between the two breaths before you begin the cycle of movement again (Figure 144).

Turning from the Inside Out

The second most essential skill in twisting is learning to initiate your twists from your inner body—that is, your organs. Review pages 64 to 70 on the organ system to refresh your memory and to help you accurately visualize the inner body. One of the most common causes of injuries in yoga practitioners is moving the musculoskeletal system farther than the underlying organs can support. If you lever your body into a twist through the dictatorial use of your arms or legs while your center remains fixed (Figure 145), there will be a conflict between your organs, which have turned one way, and your outer body, which has turned another. When both layers do not move in the same direction, the subsequent torque can cause serious strain to your joints and your spine. In all twists the muscles and bones support and *guide* the intention and initiation of the soft inner organs. In Figure 146 you can see how this person has initiated the twist from an open, turning center. Her entire body has been invited into the twist. As you move into each twist, feel whether your inner and outer body are in agreement about how far to go. Then your outer actions will always be in accord with your inner perceptions.

∾ INQUIRY ∾

Turning from the Inside Out

Sit sideways in a chair and close your eyes. Imagine your body as merely a skeleton with the pulleylike muscles attached. Begin to turn, using your arms against the back of the chair to pull yourself into the twist. Open your eyes and make a mental note of how far you could go when you used your musculoskeletal system alone. Come back to a neutral position. Close your eyes again and visualize your internal organs. Breathe into your core and dilate the organs outward. Expand your belly and, like a belly dancer, roll your belly into the twist as you exhale. Expand your stomach, liver, and spleen and, as you exhale, roll them into the twist. Working your way up the body, dilate your heart and lungs; as you exhale let them shift in the direction of the twist. Finally, visualize your soft spinal cord and adjust your bony vertebrae around the cord so that the back feels light and unrestricted. Support this inner intention with the firm guidance of your arms and legs. Now open your eyes and notice how far into the twist you have gone. Notice the difference in how you feel both physically and psychologically, practicing from the outside in and from the inside out.

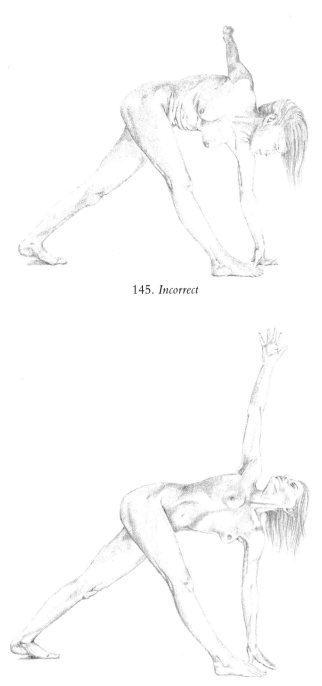

145. *Incorrect*

146. *Correct*

Cautions

Those with clinically diagnosed disc herniation should be especially cautious when practicing twists. You should be able to practice standing postures (not twisting ones), back stretches, and gentle back bends without pain before you try twisting. When you can do these movements without pain, start with standing twists, progress to reclining twists, and only when these can be done comfortably should you attempt seated twists. A safe rule of thumb is to do 50 percent of what you think you can do, then wait twenty-four hours to see what your body has to say. If you feel fine, you can progress 10 percent further, always giving yourself a day to see if there is any delayed reaction, until you are back up to your full capacity. All of this said, even two people with the same level of disc herniation will vary in their response to specific movements, with some finding great relief from twisting and others finding the slightest rotation painful. It's best not to assume that any movement will either hurt or help you but to proceed gingerly, listen intently, and follow the guidance that your body is giving you with every breath.

STANDING TWIST (page 115)

This is one of the safest ways to begin twisting, especially after recovery from a back injury. When you stand, there is less pull on your back because the hamstrings do not limit the movement of your pelvis as much as in sitting. It is therefore easier to find a neutral spinal position when standing. You can practice this casual twist frequently throughout the day to release your back before that all-too-common feeling of tension accumulates.

Crossed-Legs Twist (*Parivrtta Siddhasana*)

Here's How

This very simple twist is an ideal way to release the back, not only in your yoga practice but throughout the day whenever your back starts to feel tense. You can modify the twist and practice it in your chair at work, by simply bringing your hand onto the outside of the arm of the chair or your own thigh. This is one of the first movements I practice after intensive back bending or forward bending, to release the back.

Sit in a simple crossed-leg position, elevating your buttocks if necessary. Leading from your belly, turn to the right, bringing your hand onto the outside of your knee. On each inhalation lengthen through your torso, and on each exhalation slowly turn, working your way from the base of the spine all the way up to the head (Figure 147). Hold for thirty seconds to one minute, and then repeat on the other side. Then change the cross of the legs and repeat once more to the left and right.

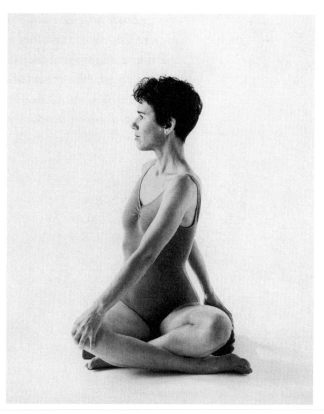

FIGURE 147

BENEFITS AND EFFECTS	Gently releases the lower back.
WHO SHOULDN'T DO THIS POSE	*See Caution above.*
PRENATAL SUGGESTIONS	

Revolved Belly Pose (*Jathara Parivartanasana*)

Here's How

Revolved Belly Pose is one of the mainstays of any yoga practice, used most frequently toward the end of a practice to release the spine and massage the internal organs before relaxation. The following three variations progress from easy to advanced.

Variation A (with support)

This is a good variation for those who are recovering from a back injury or for those with stiffness throughout the back. Lie on your back with your knees bent. Bring your knees one at a time into your chest. Inhale and, with the next exhalation, roll your knees to your right side and rest them against a pillow (Figure 148). Extend through both arms, opening the space between your shoulder blades.

Revolved Belly Pose is one posture in which you can literally "let it all hang out" to good effect. The more you can relax and breathe into the belly, the more the internal organs will be massaged and squeezed. Stay for thirty seconds to a minute. To roll to the other side, draw the left knee back to center and open it to the side until you feel the weight of the leg drawing the right leg off the floor as well. Now take the other side. If you feel very stiff, try rolling from side to side for ten brief passes before attempting to hold the pose. This will loosen the body and allow you to be more comfortable.

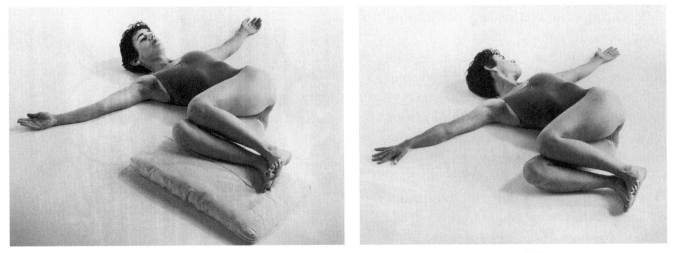

FIGURE 148   FIGURE 149

Variation B

As in the previous variation, begin by lying on your back with your knees bent and the palms facing up. With your arms extended to the sides, roll one shoulder down toward the floor so your palm turns down. Roll your other shoulder up so your palm faces up. In a very relaxed way, alternate rolling the shoulders and arms, allowing your elbows to bend slightly so the shoulders can rotate more freely.

After about ten passes, roll your knees into your chest one at a time. On your next exhalation, roll your knees to the side where the palm is facing down (Figure 149). As you change the position of your arms, roll your knees to the other side.

Continue to alternate side to side for about ten passes on each side. You may notice that your head naturally tends to turn toward the upturned palm. Let this movement happen with as little effort as possible. Notice how this exercise is initiated through the skeleton with the organs following in tow. You might imagine the bones as a washing machine agitator and the soft organs as wet, slippery clothes being moved, rolled, and turned by the action of your bones. After you have warmed your body with the rolling twists, stay for about a minute on each side.

Final Pose

Lie on the floor with your knees bent. Raise your buttocks off the floor and shift your pelvis to the left, about 6 inches off center. This little adjustment will help you to keep a neutral spinal position when you rotate to the right. Now let your knees come in toward your chest, and slowly straighten your legs. If you can't bring your legs to at least a 90-degree angle, you should continue with the bent-leg variations. On a long exhalation, lower your legs with control to the right, aim-

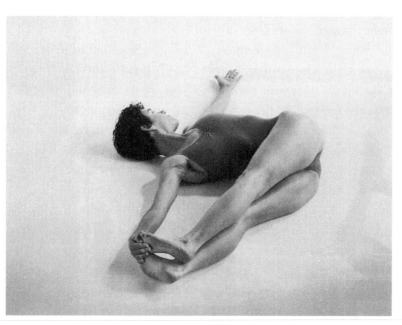

FIGURE 150

ing to bring your feet into your right hand. Release your hips away from your shoulders and broaden the space between the shoulder blades as you extend the arms strongly out to the sides (Figure 150). Stay here for a minute or more. If your abdominal and back muscles are strong, shift to the other side on an exhalation, with both legs together. Otherwise, you can bend your knees and roll one knee at a time in toward your chest. Readjust the pelvis to the right before you take the posture on the left side.

BENEFITS AND EFFECTS	Tones and stimulates the large intestine, improving elimination. Releases tension in the spinal column, hips, and shoulders. Relieves minor aches and discomfort in the lumbar spine after long sitting, forward bending, or back bending.
WHO SHOULDN'T DO THIS POSE	*See Caution above.* Those with previously dislocated hips or hip replacement prosthesis should practice with caution.
PRENATAL SUGGESTIONS	

Sage Pose I and II (*Bharadvajasana* I and II)

Here's How

Sage Pose I Kneel on a blanket and slowly let your hips slide off your heels until you are sitting to the right of your feet. Place a folded blanket underneath your right buttock until both sides of your pelvis are level. As you inhale anchor your weight through the surfaces of your body that are in contact with the floor, and as you exhale slowly turn to the right, bringing your left hand onto the outside of your right knee. Use your right hand just behind your right buttock to help maintain the lift through your back. Or, if you are stronger and more flexible, you can increase the intensity of the twist by bringing your right hand around the back of your body to take hold of your upper left arm just above the elbow (Figure 151). It's easier to take hold of the arm before your twist. Expand both shoulders out to the side as you twist, to maintain the breadth of the chest. Stay for a minute and then slowly release and repeat on the second side.

Sage Pose II In this variation you draw one leg into a Hero's Pose (page 188) and the other leg into a Half Lotus (page 152). With the left leg in a kneeling position and the right in Half Lotus, you turn to your right, reaching around your back to catch hold of the right foot. If you can't reach the foot, you can use a tie. As in the previous variation, your left hand comes onto the outside of the right knee (Figure 152). It feels particularly good if you place your left hand so the fingers

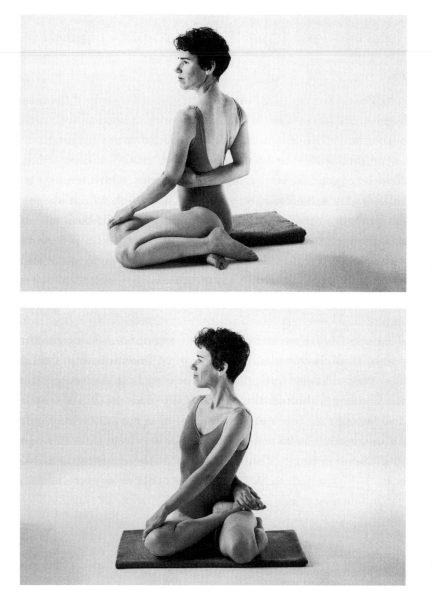

FIGURE 151

FIGURE 152

wrap around the knee to face the right hip. Then, as you turn on successive exhalations, draw the right hip out of the socket with your hand. This will create a delicious opening sensation in your hip and lower back. Stay for a minute before you change to the other side. For a particularly deep hip opener, when you complete the twist, turn to face the front and bend forward over the legs with your arms stretched in front of you.

BENEFITS AND EFFECTS	Releases the hips and lower back. Opens the shoulders, chest, and lungs. Stimulates the large and small intestines.
WHO SHOULDN'T DO THIS POSE	*See Caution above.*
PRENATAL SUGGESTIONS	Only if comfortable.

Marichi Pose I and III (*Marichyasana* I and III)

Here's How

Marichi Pose I Sit in Stick Pose, elevating your buttocks if necessary. Bend your right knee, drawing the heel of the foot toward the sitting bone on that side. On an exhalation roll your belly to the left and bring your right elbow to the inside of your knee with your hand facing upward in the "Pledge of Allegiance" position. Instead of pressing your arm against the knee, which tends to cause tension in the shoulder and back, press your knee and thigh into your arm. Gently guide your spine into the twist, working sequentially up the back until the chest has turned (Figure 153). This is the first stage of the twist. The next stage involves extending the right arm to take hold of the left foot. This gives you a little more leverage to twist but should be attempted only if you can tip forward without rounding your back. Turn your head into the twist and open your chest (Figure 154).

If you are able to turn your chest away from your leg, you are ready to try to interlock your hands. Reach your right arm around the outside of the right knee and, swinging your left arm back, take hold of your fingers. Press down through your sitting bones and through the length of the extended leg to lengthen your spine and, sustaining this length, encourage your back into a deeper rotation. Draw your arms back and down to release your shoulders away from your ears. Look back at your extended foot to create a counterrotation and release for your neck and upper back (Figure 155, shown here on the opposite side for clarity). Stay for one minute and then release.

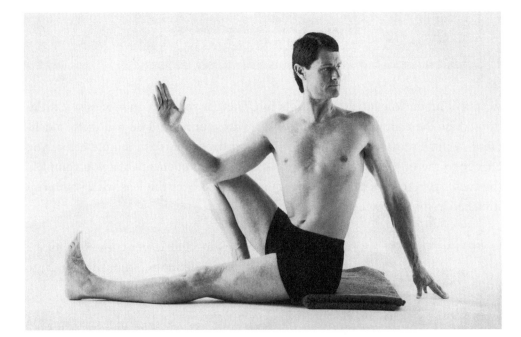

FIGURE 153

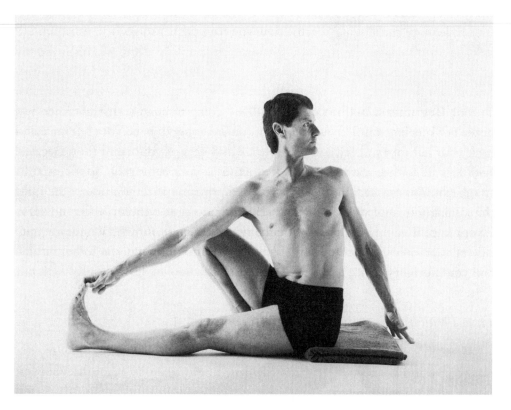

FIGURE 154

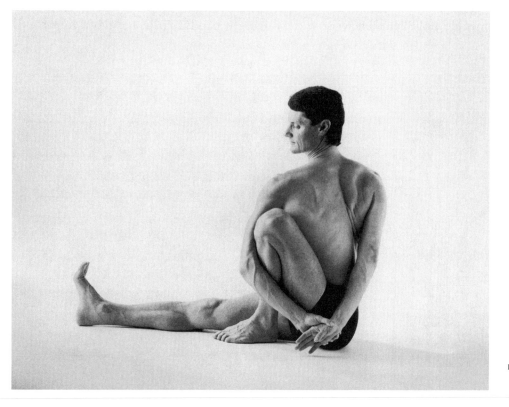

FIGURE 155

Marichi III This pose is practiced in exactly the same fashion as Marichi I, except now you bring the opposite arm to leg and turn to the *outside* of the knee. It's a little more challenging because now you have farther to go.

Variation

For Beginners: In this variation you are going to bend your right knee, but instead of keeping your left leg extended, you are going to bend your left knee and tuck your left foot in between the buttock and heel of your right foot. Because both legs are folded, you've effectively deactivated your hamstrings, so it's easier to sit upright. You can start by bringing your left arm around the outside of the right shin. Work here until your whole body is giving to the movement. When it feels as if your knee is getting in the way, you are ready to bring your elbow onto the outside of your knee. Use your other hand resting directly behind you to help maintain your upright balance (Figure 156).

Final Position

If you felt comfortable on both sides in the previous variation, now try the classic position with your left leg extended. Begin again by bringing your left elbow onto the outside of your right knee, with your left hand supporting on the floor behind you. Once your entire belly has turned toward your leg and you are able to maintain an upright position with your back, take the "hand lock" by bringing the left arm around the outside of the right shin. Link your fingers or, if possible, hold your left wrist with your right hand. Exhale and draw your hands

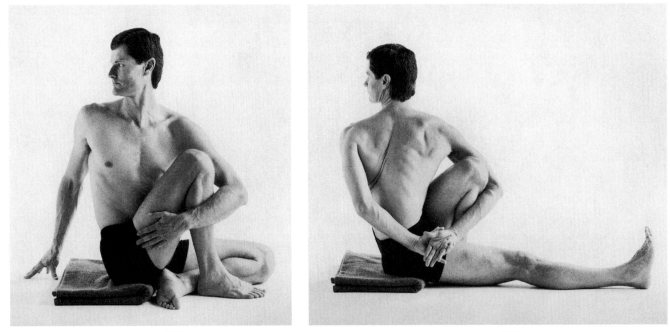

FIGURE 156   FIGURE 157

away from your shoulders, allowing the spine to lengthen strongly upward (Figure 157, shown here on opposite side for clarity).

If taking the hand lock compresses the front of the abdomen and collapses the spine, you are moving your skeleton farther than the organs can support. Go slowly and as you work into the twist, expand your organs as you inhale, direct them into the twist as you exhale, and rest in stillness in the pause in between. To complete the movement, look back toward your left foot to give your neck and upper back a deep counterrotation. Take a few more breaths and then release and repeat to the other side.

BENEFITS AND EFFECTS	Stimulates the circulation, tone, and function of the internal organs, especially the liver, lungs, and spleen. Releases deeply held tension in the back, neck, and shoulders. Assists the elimination of toxins stored in the muscle and organ tissue.
WHO SHOULDN'T DO THIS POSE	*See Caution above.*
PRENATAL SUGGESTIONS	Not Suitable.
HAVING TROUBLE?	My back tends to round and shorten as I twist.
TRY . . .	*Practice your twists with your back a few feet from a wall. Bring one arm onto the bent knee to assist the twist, and press your other arm against the wall to assist the upward movement of your back. Sit far enough away from the wall so that your arm is straight and your shoulders are relaxed.*

Lord of the Fishes Pose
(*Ardha Matsyendrasana*)

Here's How

Fold your left leg underneath you so that you are sitting on your left foot. Ideally, if you sit on the side of the foot, your left buttock will be on the side of your left heel and your right buttock will be on the side of the ball of the foot. Using your hands to assist you, draw your right leg over the left and place your right foot close to your left hip. On an inhalation lengthen through your spine, and as you exhale, roll your entire torso to the right, bringing your left arm around the outside of the right knee. Expand through your organs by breathing from deep within your core, and as you exhale progressively encourage the soft organs from your belly to your chest into the twist. Once your body has turned sufficiently, you'll be able to bring the elbow onto the outside of your right thigh. Pressing your right thigh firmly against your arm, encourage the spine to rotate farther.

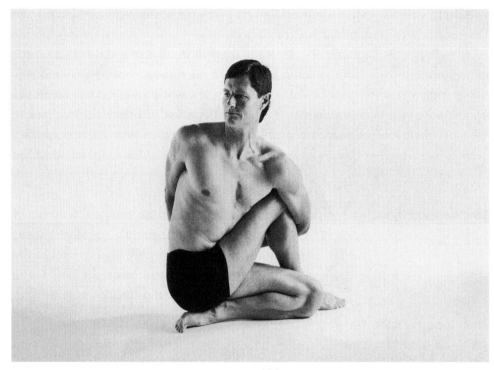

FIGURE 158

When your chest is turned to face the right leg, you are ready to try the hand interlock. For this you bring the left arm around the outside of the right thigh and shin and go around the leg to take the interlock (Figure 158). It's tempting to collapse the back to achieve this, so focus in your first few breaths on lengthening upward. Release the shoulders away from the ears and breathe as fully as you can. Stay for thirty seconds to one minute and then release. Take a moment to enjoy the sensation of fresh blood and fluid flushing through your body as you release out of the movement.

BENEFITS AND EFFECTS	Strong opener for the shoulders, upper back, and neck. Stimulates the liver, spleen, heart, and lungs. Releases built-up heat and toxins stored in the organs and tissues.
WHO SHOULDN'T DO THIS POSE	*See Caution above.*
PRENATAL SUGGESTIONS	Not Suitable.
HAVING TROUBLE?	It hurts to sit on my foot.
TRY . . .	*Until your feet and ankles become more flexible, try sitting on a folded blanket or cushion between your two feet. Raise your buttocks until your pelvis is slightly higher than the level of the underside knee. This will allow you to elongate your spine freely.*

V

The Back Bends

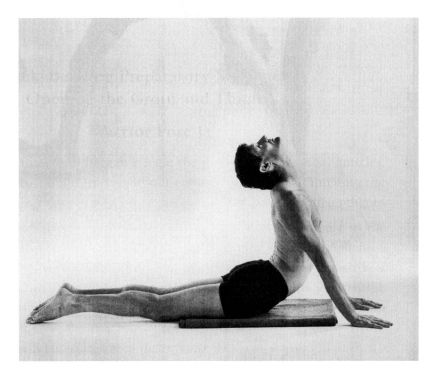

INTRODUCTION

With their emphasis on opening the heart, lungs, and chest, back bends exhilarate, bringing a sense of lightness and vitality that wards off even the most tenacious lethargy or depression. Almost all our daily activities bend the body forward, whether washing the dishes, gardening, driving to work, or typing at the computer. Over the course of years the spine can begin to round forward, causing the shoulders to hunch, the lungs to collapse, and the muscles in the back to become like tight wires as they do their best to keep this cowering structure from toppling. When we bend the spine backward, we take a defiant step away from this downward plunge, counteracting the not-so-inevitable effects of aging and in doing so giving ourselves a more "uplifted" perspective on life.

Because we rarely bend the spine into extension in our everyday activities, when you begin practicing back bends it's important to do it gradually, so your body has a chance to adjust to this new movement. In particular, you'll want to be cautious of straining your lower back and neck or overtaxing weak back muscles by doing postures that are too arduous too soon. While these movements have the potential to be powerful healers, like all strong medicine, they have the potential to be injurious if practiced without discretion. Because these postures are so impressive, it's easy to get caught up in trying to do deeper and more difficult back bends, casting caution to the breeze. So rather than measure your progress by how much you can bend your back, judge your progress in terms of how much easier it is to sit, stand, and walk with your back firmly and easily upright throughout the day. This erect carriage will impart an elegance and dignity to your entire bearing.

KEY MOVING PRINCIPLES FOR THE BACK BENDS

3. RADIATE
Move from the Inside Out: The Human Starfish

4. CENTER
Maintain the Integrity of the Spine: The Central Axis

7. ENGAGE
Use the Whole Body: Review the Organs and Glands

ESSENTIAL SKILLS

Elongate Before Bending Backward

～ *Using the Whole Spine: Mobilizing the Upper Back*

When you bend backward you want to distribute the extension as evenly as possible throughout the length of your back. This would be easy to do if all parts of the vertebral column had an equal capacity for extension. Unfortunately, the thoracic spine, which tends to become the most stiff and most rounded, is also the least able to extend. Left to its own devices the body will choose the easiest option available to it, so that when you bend backward all the movement centers around the lower back and neck—just where the back is most vulnerable. In this first section you'll learn why this is so and what to do to protect your back, opening the tighter areas that tend to accumulate tension while strengthening the more vulnerable parts of your spine.

Girded by the ribs and limited in movements of extension by the shape and angle of its joint surfaces, the thoracic spine is an inherently more rigid part of the back than the structures above and below it—the neck and lower back. The spinous processes in the neck and lower back are relatively stubby, allowing for often extreme ranges of forward and backward movement. While elongation is the precursor movement for *any* action in the spine, it is particularly important in the thoracic spine, because the spinous processes in this area of the back are very long. You can see that it does not take very much backward motion before these processes wedge against each other and prevent further motion (Figure 160a). If,

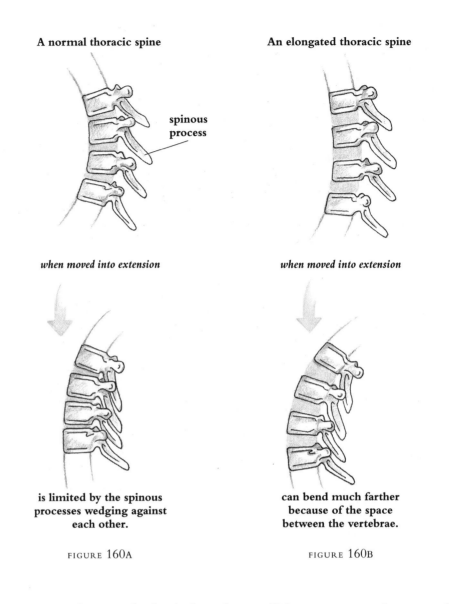

A normal thoracic spine

An elongated thoracic spine

spinous
process

when moved into extension

when moved into extension

**is limited by the spinous
processes wedging against
each other.**

**can bend much farther
because of the space
between the vertebrae.**

FIGURE 160A

FIGURE 160B

however, you elongate the back first, there will be more space between the processes, and hence more ease in going farther backward without restriction (Figure 160b).

～ INQUIRY ～

Elongating the Spine Before Extension

As you are sitting in your chair, experiment by bringing your head and neck into extension, focusing on the back-bending action alone. Go only as far as you can without discomfort. Make a mental note of the place on the wall or ceiling where your gaze fell, which marks your fullest degree of extension.

Now come back into a neutral position. Begin the movement this time by pressing down through your sitting bones and legs and reaching up through the top of your head. Concentrate on the upward movement of elongation as if you were bending back over a huge ball and wanted to avoid touching it. Do not allow your neck to collapse backward but maintain the upward lift through your neck by keeping your gaze low. Each time you inhale, go up, and as you exhale, begin to arc slightly backward without losing the reaching action through your back. Again, go only as far as you can without discomfort. Notice whether you can go farther backward when you support the movement by elongating throughout the action. Did your second attempt feel more comfortable?

MOBILIZING THE RIGID AREAS OF THE BACK— BALANCING THE ACTION THROUGHOUT THE BODY

While it is important to focus on opening the thoracic spine in back bends, it's also equally important to support the action of extension with your whole body. In particular, you'll want to warm and loosen your shoulders and groin before practicing back bends. The shoulders, neck, and upper back work in synchrony, and when the shoulders become tight, this impacts the ability of the other areas to move effectively. Additionally, when you bend back- ward, and the front of the groin and upper thighs do not give to the action, you will tend to seesaw on your lower back, causing compres- sion in this area (Figure 161). Notice how the person with open groin and shoulders can extend his whole body in a smooth, continuous arc (Figure 162), while the person inflexible in these areas hinges all the action in the lower back. The preparatory stretches that begin on page 180 are wonderful for opening all these areas. You can use them not only to prepare for back bends but as part of your regular practice routine. By following this section carefully, you'll learn to loosen the tighter segments of your back while keeping your neck and lower back healthy.

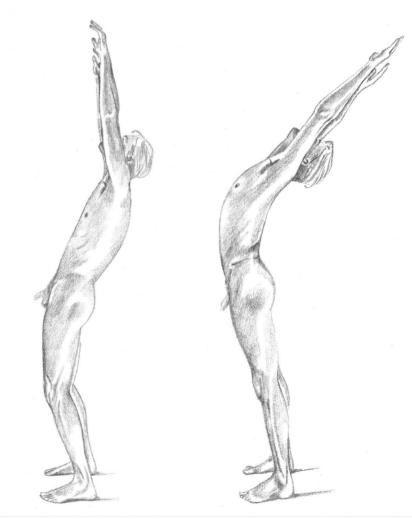

FIGURE 161. *Incorrect*   FIGURE 162. *Correct*

Support Your Back from the Front

~ *The Hyoid: The Keystone of Upright Posture*

In our development as human beings the tonification of our digestive tract precedes the use and initiation of movement through our spinal column. This concept may at first be difficult to grasp if you think of your spine as being supported entirely by the action of your muscles. The long period in which we breast-feed as infants not only nourishes us but increases the tone throughout the digestive tract from mouth to anus, preparing us for when we'll need to connect our head through our spine to our tail. In sucking and swallowing we create a "firmness" along the entire length of the digestive tract, and this soft vertical axis will act as a support for the front of the spine. When you sit, stand, or move your back against gravity (as when you come up in the Cobra Pose), both the front and back of your body must participate in the movement. Many of us have forgotten how to engage this inner organic support in our bodies. To find this support for the back, we have to reawaken neurological connections that produce an efficient pattern of whole-body movement. This approach is very different from the modern (and usually unsuccessful) approaches to back care, which use reductionistic strategies of strengthening isolated muscle groups such as the abdominal or thigh muscles, rather than the functional use of the whole body in integrated action.

One of the most helpful keystones in eliciting this crucial support for the spine lies in the positioning of a hidden bone in your body—the hyoid (pronounced *hi-oid*) (Figure 163). Your entire digestive and respiratory systems are suspended energetically from this one keystone.[1] Like the psoas muscles that connect and integrate the lower spine with the pelvis and legs, the hyoid is the bridge between your head and neck and your upper torso (Figure 164).

To appreciate the hyoid's role in the body, it is necessary to understand the most salient points of its anatomy. Located in the upper front part of the neck, this small U-shaped bone serves as a point of attachment for the muscles located in the floor of the mouth and tongue and for muscles that extend below the bone. Suspended by ligaments from the styloid process of the temporal bone, it has the curious distinction of being the only bone in the body that does not articulate (form a joint) with any other bone.

Mirroring the psoas, the hyoid muscles traverse the hyoid bone and create a bridge that connects the base of the skull and the floor of the mouth with the sternum in the front of the body and the tip of the scapula in the back. Anatomically it's very complex, so for the sake of simplicity, let's focus on function.

When the hyoid bone moves back and up toward the front of your cervical vertebrae (as in sucking or swallowing), it provokes a response throughout the digestive tract, causing it to tone and lengthen parallel to your spine. Simultaneously the abdominal muscles move in and up. The hyoid also mechanically lifts the breastbone toward the chin, since the sternohyoid muscles insert on the inside of the upper tip of the sternum. The heart and lungs lift, the belly organs increase in

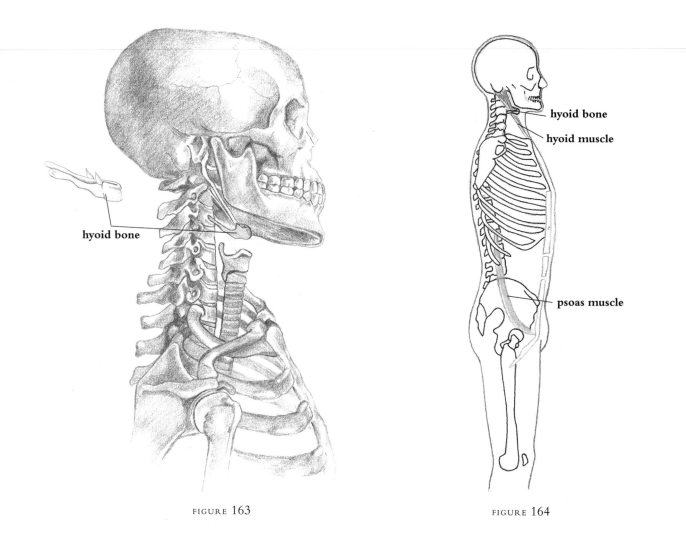

FIGURE 163   FIGURE 164

tone, and quite miraculously the front of the body now begins to share the role of supporting the spinal column. When the hyoid bone drops down and forward and the chin juts up and out, the cervical and lumbar spine respond by collapsing and curving forward, while the abdominal wall becomes lax. You can now begin to see how the supporting action that is elicited through the engagement of the hyoid contributes to erect carriage of the whole body. It's more important that you feel this action. Try the following inquiry.

～ INQUIRY ～

Engaging the Hyoid

Sit comfortably in a chair and place one hand on your belly and one hand on your breastbone. Placing your hands in these areas will help you gauge the effects of the hyoid's position. Start by dropping your throat forward, letting the chin jut out and up (Figure 165a). Notice how the belly collapses downward and out and how the breastbone, heart, and lungs sink within the chest. The digestive tract becomes slack. Notice that once you've collapsed through the hyoid and thrown your head back, it's almost impossible to lift your chest. Now inhale and draw the front of the throat back toward the neck, and lift your sternum. Draw the chin down onto the chest, lengthening the back of the neck. (Figure 165b). Notice that as you strongly engage the action of the hyoid, the abdomen has become long and lean and the chest is now buoyant. And, now that the thoracic spine is supporting the action, if you choose to bring your head back in extension, the movement will feel comfortable as the action is distributed throughout the upper spine and neck. If your breastbone is vertical, try bringing your head back, and notice how different this is compared to when you brought the head and neck back as an isolated movement.

You may find it helpful to imagine your chest as a ball, and your head and neck as another ball stacked one over the other, like a snowman. In the collapsing action the balls revolve away from each other, and in the lifting action they revolve toward each other.

Now find a position between these two extremes where the hyoid moves slightly in, up, and back toward the neck without undue tension in the throat. Your eyes will be level with the horizon as you release the base of the skull lightly upward (Figure 165c). Feel how engaging the action of the hyoid is giving the spine support just where it needs it—your lower back and neck. This engagement should precede bringing the head back as is done in many of the more advanced back bends.

Now it's time to see how to integrate this into your back bending! Most people begin a back bend by thrusting the chin forward and up and hinging on the neck. This action tells the organs of the trunk to collapse forward and away from the spine, so that not only are they not helping the spine, they are hanging as dead

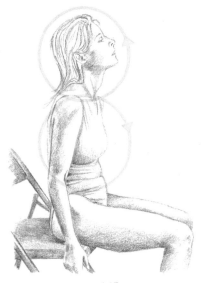
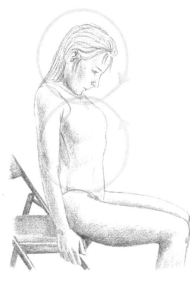
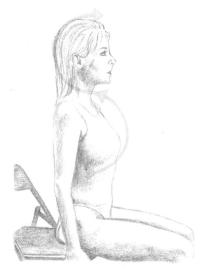

FIGURE 165A   FIGURE 165B   FIGURE 165C

weights from the now overtaxed back muscles. To integrate this awareness into your practice of extension, try this simple exercise. If you already have a back injury, do not do the beginning of this inquiry (the wrong way) but skip to the later part of the section.

～ INQUIRY ～

Back Bending with Frontal Support

Lie facedown on the floor with a blanket folded underneath your hips and with your arms down by your sides. Sense and feel your inner organs, imagining the long digestive tract that lies parallel to your spine. Begin your back bend by jutting the throat forward and lifting the chin. Try to come up off the floor initiating the movement from the forward thrust of your throat and neck. Notice how the forward position of the hyoid is setting off a cascade effect, causing the organs to collapse down and away from the spinal column. Feel how the neck and lower back compress and the breastbone drops. When you come up like this, it's impossible to lift the breastbone and engage the action of the thoracic spine. All the action is in the neck and lower back (Figure 166a). Come down and rest. Now, by keeping the

chin level and your gaze low, imagine your inner organs expanding up into your spine, then as you exhale, draw the hyoid in and up, feeling for the inner support of your organs as you lift the head, neck, and chest off the floor (Figure 166b). Could you come up higher as you engaged the frontal support for your spine? Fantastic. Now you are ready to begin your practice of these enlivening movements.

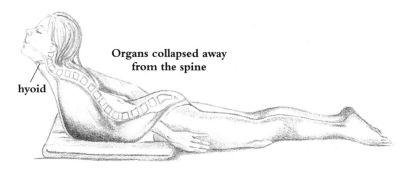

FIGURE 166A. *Incorrect*

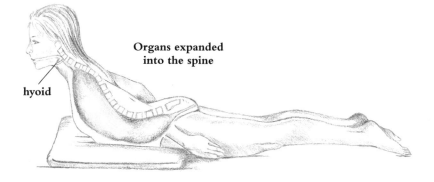

FIGURE 166B. *Correct*

Back-Bending Preparatory Stretches:
Opening the Shoulders

The Shoulder Clock

Here's How

Stand at a right angle to a wall with your right shoulder facing the wall. Check that your feet are hips-width apart so you'll have a solid foundation underneath you. Stand about 8 inches away from the wall. Depending on your flexibility, you can move closer to the wall, which will make the exercise more challenging, or as far away as a foot or more, which will make it easier. Extend your arm up the wall like the hand of a clock pointing to twelve. Take a moment to press down through your heels and to relax your neck and jaw. After several breath cycles, extend the arm back to one o'clock. Keep reaching the arm as high as you can up the wall. Again stay for several breaths and continue moving through the imaginary digits of the clock face until you reach three o'clock (Figure 167). As you come to three o'clock, lean your chest forward slightly, turning your breastbone toward the center of the room. You'll feel a strong opening in the front of your chest and shoulder, an area that can become chronically tight through slouching. Take several breaths here and then let your arm swing down to your side. Stand for a moment and feel the difference between the two arms. If you look in a mirror, you may be able to see that one arm is longer than the other. The extra length is simply a measure of how much you have released the arm out of the shoulder socket. Repeat the shoulder clock on the other side. If you have time, return to the first side and do the exercise standing a little closer to the wall.

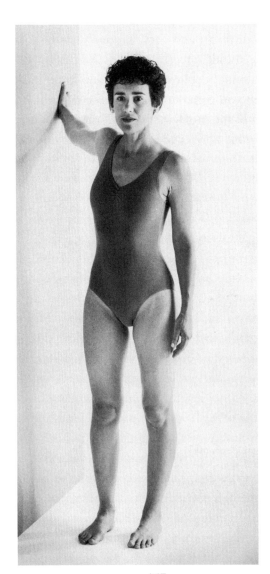

FIGURE 167

Shoulder Chair Stretch

You'll Need

A clear wall space and a chair

Here's How

This is a great movement for releasing and opening the shoulder joints and the front of the chest. Place a chair against the wall with the seat facing you. Come into a kneeling position in front of the chair, and place your elbows shoulder-width apart on the edge of the seat. Let your weight rest on the *outer* edge of your elbows rather than the inner edge, so that your shoulder girdle broadens out to the sides. Rest your forehead on the edge of the seat and press the fingertips together over your head in a prayer position. Walk your knees back until they are directly under your hips. Expand your breath into your upper chest, back, and shoulders, pressing the elbows firmly downward as you reach back through your hips. Feel your armpits lengthening, and with each breath allow your upper back to release downward (Figure 168). Stay for as long as you feel comfortable, gradually deepening the intensity of the opening. When you've had enough, slowly walk your knees in toward your arms until you can take your elbows off the chair. Rest for a few moments in a kneeling position, enjoying the sensation of your now opened chest and shoulders. Is it easier to breathe?

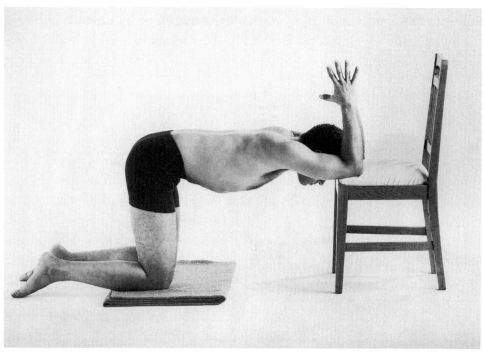

FIGURE 168

Back-Bending Preparatory Stretches: Opening the Back

The use of yoga props is particularly helpful when you are trying to open specific segments of your back. Take time experimenting with how best to use the props for your particular structure. Your back will thank you for this small investment of time by giving you hours of ease and lightness later.

Back Bend over a Bolster: Opening the Upper Back

You'll Need

A bolster or 2 or 3 blankets

Here's How

This movement opens the upper back into extension while expanding the heart and lungs and freeing the breath.

Sit on the floor with your knees bent in front of you. Place a rolled-up blanket or bolster under your knees. Roll a second blanket into a tight cylinder and place it directly behind you on the floor. Bring your elbows to rest on the roll and slowly recline over the roll so that it crosses your body at the level of your mid–shoulder blades (nipple line). Roll up one end of a blanket and wedge it underneath your neck so that the curve of your neck is completely supported. Now extend your arms with the elbows bent over the head. The body should cascade evenly over the rolls—if you feel discomfort at any point in the back, adjust the size and position of the rolls (Figure 169). If you can't release the shoulders onto the floor without creating an uncomfortable arch in your neck, you probably need to reduce the diame-

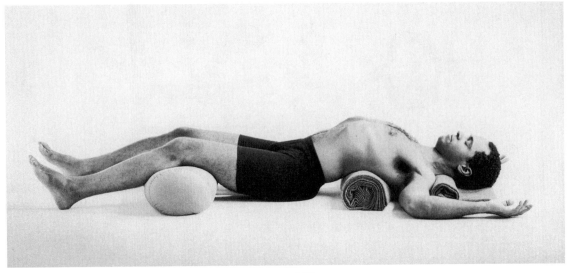

FIGURE 169

ter of the bolster (try about 6 inches). Stay here for about three to seven minutes, letting the body become accustomed to the opening. If you would like to increase the intensity of the opening, remove the roll from under your neck and extend your arms over your head along the floor. At the same time extend the legs until they are completely straight. In this final position the upper back and shoulders receive a strong opening. After you have stayed in the pose for a few minutes, feel free to experiment with your positioning by placing the bolster a little higher or lower under your back. Rather than move the bolster, it is better to bend your knees and scoot toward your head or feet before lying back again.

This stretch can be very intense the first time, so don't stay too long. When you're ready to come out, bend your knees and roll onto your side. Never try to come out of the position by sitting up. Relax on your side before coming to a sitting position. When you sit up, notice whether it is easier to be upright after opening the spine into extension. After a while this upright stance will feel "normal," and slouching will feel uncomfortable and tiring.

Back Bend Through a Chair

You'll Need

A metal folding chair
A clear wall space
A yoga mat
A bolster or stack of pillows

Here's How

These movements help you to open selectively the thoracic spine, chest, and shoulders while keeping your neck and lower back relatively neutral.

Variation A

Find a sturdy folding chair with a wide opening between the seat and back of the chair. Fold your yoga sticky mat and place it along the edge of the chair for padding. Position the chair a few feet away from a wall with the back facing the wall. Have a bolster close at hand. Straddle the chair and climb your legs through the opening between the seat and the back. Now begin to recline back and, as you do so, slide your buttocks through the chair until your upper back is resting on the edge of the chair (about nipple line). Bring your hands behind your head to support your neck, and slowly recline over the edge of the chair. If you have a bolster or a stack of pillows, place these under your head (Figure 170). This support will allow you to keep your head and neck in a neutral position while you focus on opening your chest, shoulders, and upper back. Make sure that you have not moved so far through the chair that you are now bending from the base of your ribs and your waist rather than through the thoracic part of your back.

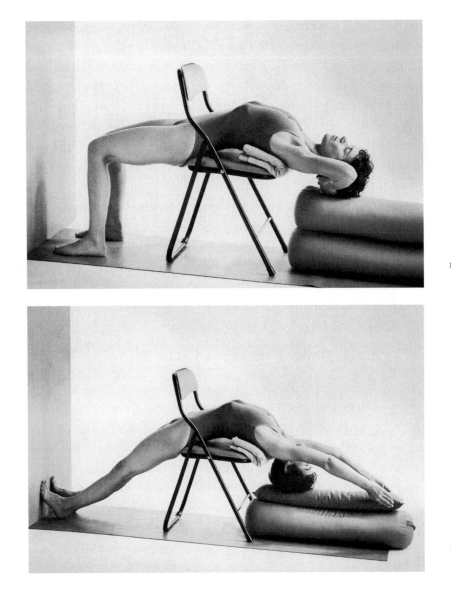

FIGURE 171

If you are feeling comfortable, you can deepen the degree of extension. Slowly extend your legs, pressing strongly through your feet and reaching your tail away from your head. Press your feet into the wall in front of the chair, readjusting the position of the chair if need be. Reach your arms over your head and, if you are able, grasp the end of the bolster (Figure 171). This will intensify the opening in your shoulders and upper back. Stay for a minute or more, breathing deeply. To come out of the position, bend your knees, bring your hands onto the seat of the chair, and slowly draw yourself up. Rest, letting your body fold over the back of the chair. When you come back up to sitting, feel how erect and light your posture is after this deep movement.

Variation B
This variation is particularly good for people who have hypermobile lower backs that tend to bend excessively from the base of the rib cage. Place your chair

on a sticky mat so it is secure, and pad the edge with a second mat or folded towel and place a small pillow on the seat of the chair. This will be used to support your head later. Sit on the floor facing away from the seat of the chair. Lifting your buttocks off the floor, carefully bring your elbows onto the seat of the chair. Place your upper back along the edge of the chair and slowly slide backward until you can reach your arms through the gap between the seat and the back of the chair. If this is too intense for your shoulders, you can simply bend your elbows and grasp the back of the seat of the chair. Otherwise, reach your arms through the gap and straighten them

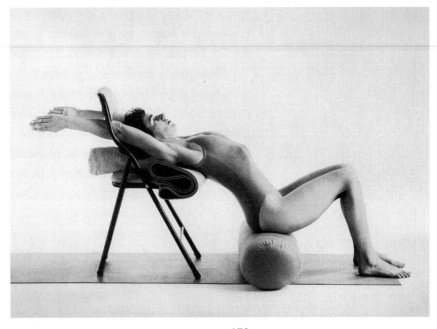

FIGURE 172

completely. You'll want to support your neck and head with the pillow so you can focus on releasing your upper back alone. Now, *very* slowly, begin to hinge from your upper back, drawing your lower ribs down toward your belly and lowering your buttocks toward the floor. You can place a bolster under your buttocks or, if you are more flexible, you can bring your buttocks all the way to the floor (Figure 172). This will depend on your back and shoulder flexibility and to some degree your body proportions. Don't strain, and go slowly. You'll no doubt be getting in touch with some very tight places in your back and shoulders. Breathe fully into these places in your body, and exhale completely, allowing yourself to sigh out through your mouth. As you become more familiar with the action, you can experiment by shifting up or down the thoracic spine to mobilize specific segments. Stay for one to three minutes and, when you release, take a few moments to feel the effects of this dramatic opening.

Back Bend over a Ball

You'll Need

A 24″, 29″, or 34″ Gymnic Ball (see page 28)

Here's How

I do not usually include work that requires specialized equipment, but these balls are so incredible for releasing tension in the back in a safe and pleasurable way that I would recommend any serious practitioner invest in one. They can be used not only for your yoga practice but as wonderful chairs. I keep one in my office for regular back releases in between long hours at the computer.

Place your ball on top of your yoga mat so it will not slip. With the ball behind you, bend your knees and rest your hands on the ball to give you support as you recline back. Slowly roll headward over the ball, making small rocking motions back and forth between your head and feet. The more you move toward your head, the more challenging it will be for your back, and the more you move toward your feet, the easier it will be for your back. As you feel confident, reach

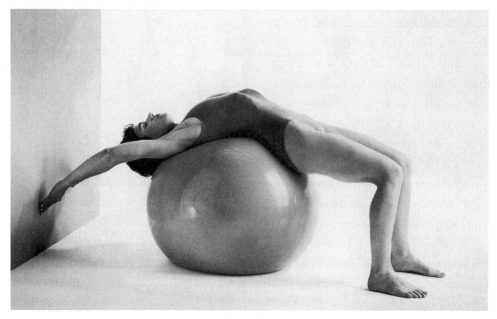

FIGURE 173

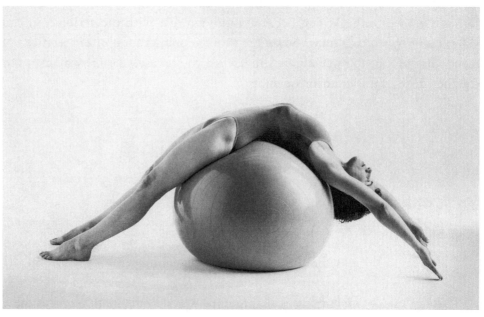

FIGURE 174

your arms over your head. Notice that you have to work evenly or you'll roll off the ball. For security you can place a wall behind you or have a friend watch you the first time (Figure 173). Also, if your upper back is very stiff, you'll find that your head and neck are arching backward with your chin up. Use a folded blanket to lift the head until your neck feels absolutely relaxed. If you want to deepen the opening in your back, straighten your legs slowly, reaching through your heels to keep the length in your lower back. Eventually you'll be able to touch your hands to the floor with your back in a deep arc (Figure 174). To come out of the movement, gently rock toward your feet until you are in the squatting start position. You can rest the ball against a wall and lean against it as you squat and release your back the other way.

Back-Bending Preparatory Stretches: Opening the Groin and Thighs

Warrior Pose I

Any lunging movement will help to release the groin and deep psoas muscles, allowing the back to extend freely without compression. You can intensify the lunge of Warrior I by drawing your hips close to the floor and then attempting to straighten your leg *without* lifting your hips away from the floor (Figure 175). You may be unable to straighten your leg very far, but that is unimportant. If you feel a deep opening in the front of the left groin, the stretch is working.

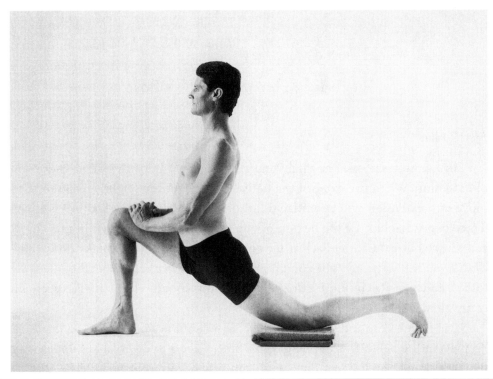

FIGURE 175

Hero's Pose and Reclining Hero/Heroine's Pose
(*Virasana* and *Supta Virasana*)

You'll Need

> 3 or 4 blankets
> A bolster
> 1 sandbag or a bag of rice

Hero's Pose (Preparatory Position)

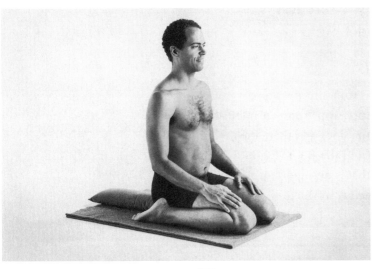

FIGURE 176

From a kneeling position lift your buttocks off your heels and place them instead in between your feet on the floor. Draw your calf muscles outward with a spreading action of your thumbs, and extend your toes directly behind you. If sitting on the floor is uncomfortable in your knees or the tops of your feet, raise your buttocks onto a narrowly folded blanket or bolster (Figure 176). As your quadriceps release you can gradually reduce the height of your seat until you can sit with ease directly on the floor. You should be able to sit this way comfortably before proceeding to the next variations.

Reclining Hero/Heroine's Pose

Here's How

These postures release the thighs and groin so they can participate in the action of extension. When the front of the body has become very tight, any attempt to move into extension will be initiated through the lumbar spine and pelvis alone. These two variations use the flexion of one leg to prevent the pelvis from arching, and thus stabilize the lower back while giving you access to those pesky groin muscles. If you feel discomfort or compression in your lower back when both legs are folded under in Reclining Hero, these variations should eliminate the problem completely.

Sit in Hero's Pose and extend your left leg forward in front of you on the floor. To prevent the pelvis from tipping to the side, place a folded blanket under your left buttock until both sides of the pelvis are even. Secure your other leg by placing a sandbag on the thigh—this will help you anchor the leg so you can deepen the opening in the groin. Now slowly recline back onto your elbows, drawing the base of your rib cage onto the floor first, then releasing your whole torso to the floor. If coming all the way to the floor creates a deep arc in your lower back, raise your back onto an angled bolster (Figure 177). Press through the heel of the left leg as you draw the tail under to bring the pelvis into a neutral position. Extend your arms over your head and reach through the back of your hands. This action will intensify the sensation along the top of the right leg and into the groin and lower abdomen. Stay for one to three minutes, then repeat on the other side.

If you felt comfortable with the previous variation, return to the first side, except this time draw your left knee in toward your chest (Figure 178). By drawing your knee into the chest, you will be flexing the pelvis and lumbar against the extension of the bent leg. To deepen the opening, press the top of the right foot into the floor, an action that will lower the right hip closer to the floor. Stay for one to three minutes, then repeat on the other side.

Final Position

As you become more flexible you'll be able to practice the posture with your buttocks on the floor and without support behind you. Sit in Hero's Pose. As you begin to lean back, actively draw the coccyx under and let the abdomen draw back toward the spine, using the support of your arms. Go slowly so you can maintain parallel legs and ensure that the knees stay on the floor. Lower the base of your rib cage onto the floor first, then continue to recline until the whole torso is lying on the floor. Actively elongate the sitting bones toward the backs of the knees so the pelvis is kept in a neutral position. Then reach the arms over the head, reaching through the backs of the hands so the spine grows long and relaxed (Figure 179).

Reclining Hero is not a back bend but an opening for the front of the groin and thighs.

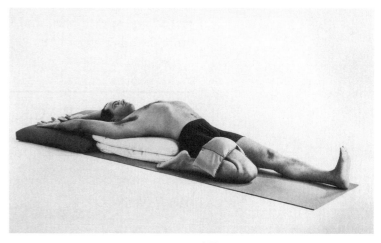

FIGURE 177

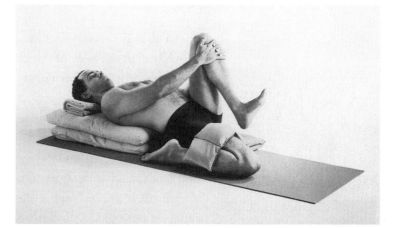

FIGURE 178

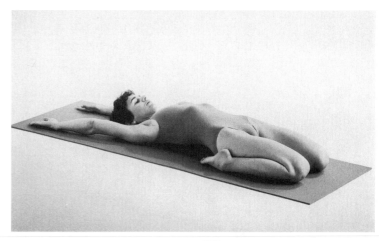

FIGURE 179

The lower rib cage should be in contact with the floor, and the lumbar curve should not be exaggerated. A small gap between the lumbar spine and the floor is normal, but this gap should not be pronounced. If it is, you are probably not ready to assume the full position and should lie against an angled bolster. Any pain in the lower back is a sure sign that you are compressing the back rather than lengthening through it. After you have practiced Reclining Hero, straighten both legs completely and stretch back into Downward-Facing Dog (page 116) to release the groin the other way.

THE BACK-BENDING POSTURES

Locust Pose (*Salabhasana*)

You'll Need

　2 blankets

Here's How

In all these variations raise your hips and pelvis on a folded blanket. Your hips should be on the edge of the blanket, with the thighs off. This will help to decrease the angle of the lumbar curve. Some people find two blankets give them greater ease.

Variation A

One of the gentlest ways to begin with the practice of Locust is with the arms and legs spread wide apart so the body forms a starfish shape. Imagine your limbs (head, tail, arms, and legs) as fluid projections from your navel center. Raising the left arm and right leg acts to counterbalance the weight through the spine, making this variation an excellent way to start if you have a weak back.

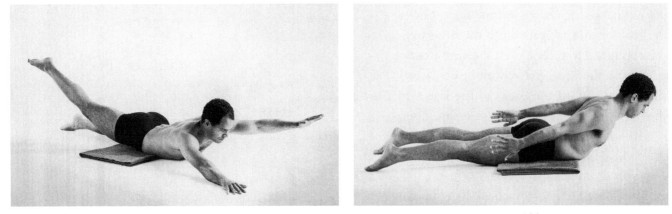

FIGURE 180　　　　　　　　　　　　　　　FIGURE 181

Lie with your hips raised slightly on a folded blanket and stretch your right leg and left arm away from each other without raising them off the floor. Wait until you can feel a tautness through your center. As you feel the connection between your center and your opposing limbs, slowly raise them an inch off the floor, allowing your head, neck, and chest to come up lightly. Resist the temptation to initiate the movement by raising your head and chin—keep the gaze low and the neck long, focusing on using your back muscles evenly (Figure 180). In this way you will be strengthening your back muscles in a lengthened position. As you lower your limbs, reach them farther out, grasping the floor with your fingers. You'll now feel very long across one diagonal. Proceed to the second side. Work through each diagonal several times, letting the limbs come higher off the ground as you feel the center opening and releasing. Then rest in Child's Pose (page 193) to release your back.

Variation B

Place your arms by your sides with your palms facing your thighs and the fingers stretched back toward your feet. Visualize your soft internal axis, your digestive tract, and its position parallel to your spinal column. Imagine lifting yourself up like a caterpillar, drawing your front body up into your back body. On your next exhalation, slowly come up off the floor, reaching your arms back toward your feet. It's essential to keep the head and neck in a neutral position. Take three breaths in and out, raising yourself a little higher on each successive exhalation, drawing the organs of your front body up into your back body (Figure 181). Feel the connection from your mouth all the way through to your anus and how this internal energetic line mirrors the connection between your hard skull, vertebral column, and your tail. On your next exhalation slowly come down. Repeat three times and then rest in Child's Pose.

Variation C

Lying facedown, bring your hands underneath your hips and thighs with your palms facing upward. As you breathe out, lengthen your legs away from your

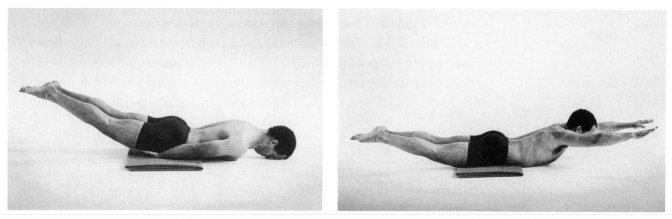

FIGURE 182   FIGURE 183

center and slowly draw your right leg up off the floor. Take about three breaths as you reach the leg out of your belly. Then slowly lower and repeat on the left side. If these variations were comfortable for you, on your next exhalation, raise both legs simultaneously, concentrating on lengthening through your body rather than lifting your legs high off the floor (Figure 182). Stay for about three breaths, maintaining the length through your center, and then release. Repeat this variation three times before relaxing in Child's Pose.

Final Position

In this final variation both arms and legs come up off the floor. The farther you extend your arms and legs away from your center, the greater the stress on the core back muscles. The traditional way of lifting the arms and legs from a straightened position is a dead lift for the back—the equivalent of lifting a heavy parcel while holding it a few feet from your trunk. In this variation you'll gradually straighten your arms, thereby gradually increasing the work of the back muscles.

Begin lying on your belly with your arms extended out to the sides. Slowly raise your arms and chest off the floor. Bend your elbows to form a right angle between the lower and upper arm. Now here comes the challenging part: Slowly tip your elbows downward as you raise your forearms and point them upward at a slight angle. Check that there is a straight line between your forearm and hand, because it's common for people simply to flex at the wrists rather than rotate the shoulder back. When you tip the elbows correctly, you'll feel the muscles at the base of your shoulder blades working strongly. These muscles draw the shoulder blades down so that you can stand with your back upright.

Now begin to slowly straighten your arms on successive exhalations, following the angle of your forearms up and out. As you do so, begin to lift both of your legs off the floor, opening the legs and arms away from your navel center. Explore where you feel the clearest connection between your navel, head, tail, arms, and legs (Figure 183). If at any point your lower back muscles signal that they have reached their maximum, then stay at a point just before you feel potential strain. For some people that will mean the arms will only half straighten. Don't worry about how far you go, because if you work correctly with what you can do today, you are building a pathway to the final variation. Stay for one to three breaths and, as you come down, reach the arms and legs farther out along the floor. Grasp the fingers against the floor as you come down, pressing your pubic bone into the floor to give your lower back an extra release. Repeat this variation one to three times, then rest in Child's Pose or practice Downward-Facing Dog (page 116).

BENEFITS AND EFFECTS   Strengthens the back muscles and reduces kyphosis (excessive curvature of the thoracic spine). Improves erect carriage of the body. Stimulates the sex glands and reduces gas in the lower abdomen.

WHO SHOULDN'T DO THIS POSE	Those with spondylolisthesis or spondylolysis should practice Locust only with the assistance of an experienced teacher.
PRENATAL SUGGESTIONS	Not suitable.
HAVING TROUBLE?	My lower back is very weak, and it feels painful when I come up off the floor.
TRY ...	*Practice the variations, keeping your limbs on the floor or just slightly off the floor. Concentrate on lengthening the limbs out from your back. This action will gradually strengthen the back. Also work on strengthening your back through the regular practice of standing postures.*

Child's Pose (*Balasana*)

Here's How

Child's Pose is a great resting posture in between other postures, but especially after back bends. It releases the hips and lower back, while allowing the arms, head, and neck to rest. As it compresses the abdomen, it is also an excellent posture for alleviating gas and bloating.

Sit in a kneeling position and simply fold forward and rest your head on the floor with your arms resting on the floor alongside your heels (Figure 184). If your hips or knees are very tight and your buttocks remain raised in the air, try placing a blanket or bolster under your buttocks and a folded blanket under your forehead. Breathe low and slow, allowing your breath to massage your entire body.

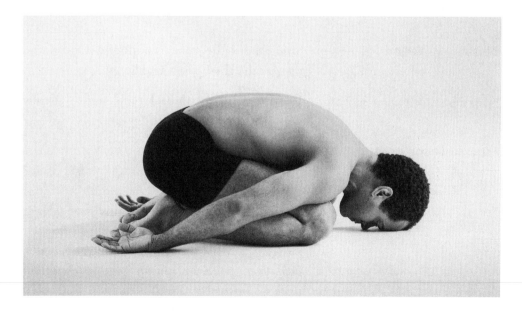

FIGURE 184

Bridge Pose (*Setu Bandhasana*)

Here's How

Lie on your back with your knees bent. Starting with your tail, begin to peel the spine off the floor, vertebra by vertebra, until your weight is resting on your shoulders. Press down firmly with your feet as you lift and draw your buttocks under toward the backs of the knees. As you look down your body, check that your thighs are parallel and your knees have not dropped outward. If you are new to the movement, simply reach your arms toward your feet. To intensify the action of this pose interlock your fingers and press your arms firmly into the floor to help you lift the chest (Figure 185). More advanced students can reach back and hold on to the ankles. Take a few breaths in your final position, and then slowly roll down through the back and rest on the floor.

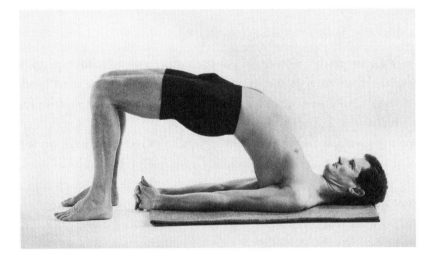

FIGURE 185

BENEFITS AND EFFECTS	Strengthens the back and thighs. Opens and releases the chest, heart, and lungs.
WHO SHOULDN'T DO THIS POSE	☺ (Even those with back problems can usually do modified versions of this position.)
PRENATAL SUGGESTIONS	
HAVING TROUBLE?	My lower back hurts.
TRY . . .	*Lift the spine only a few inches off the floor, focusing on the elongation of the back rather than the height of the position. Make sure your navel is lower than your pubic bone to ensure you are not hyperextending through your lumbar.*

Bow Pose (*Dhanurasana*)

You'll Need

2 blankets
Possibly a yoga tie

Here's How

Variation: Half Bow   Lie with your belly on a folded blanket. Without losing the length in your lower back and hips, slowly bend your right knee and reach back to take hold of the ankle with your right hand. If you can't reach the ankle comfortably, use a yoga tie wrapped around your ankle. Extend your left arm forward on the floor as a counterbalance. As you exhale, reach your right foot away from your calf (do not draw the foot toward you, as this will compress the back and shoulder). Make sure that as you reach back you are keeping the right hip on the floor. Simultaneously raise your chest off the floor with the slight assistance of your left arm (Figure 186). Stay for three to five breaths, gradually opening the thigh, groin, and back of your bent leg.

Final Position

In the Full Bow you begin in the same way, only now you'll bend both knees and clasp your ankles with both hands. As you exhale, reach your feet back and away from your shoulders, raising your knees and chest off the floor (Figure 187). Resist the temptation to throw your head back. Instead, concentrate on raising your breastbone up to a vertical position. Bow Pose can be done in many ways, depending on how you want to work your body. You can rock your weight toward your knees, bringing your legs low and your chest high, or you can raise the knees and shoulders evenly. Experiment with where you feel the most satisfying stretch. Stay for three to five breaths, and then release the legs and rest on the floor. Repeat several times before resting in Child's Pose.

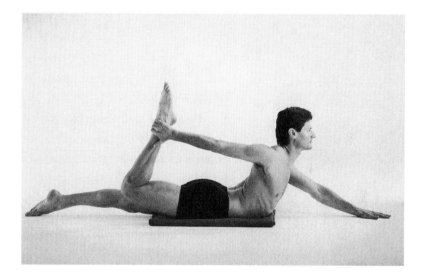

FIGURE 186

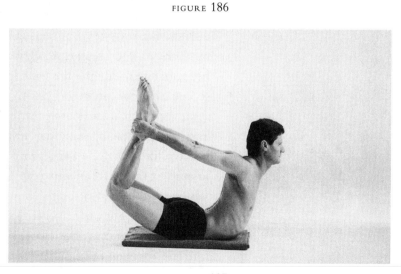

FIGURE 187

BENEFITS AND EFFECTS	Strengthens the entire back and releases the thighs and groin. Opens and releases the chest, heart, and lungs. Reduces the buildup of heat in the internal organs.
WHO SHOULDN'T DO THIS POSE	Those with spondylolisthesis or spondylolysis should practice Bow only with the assistance of an experienced teacher. Those with knee injuries should be cautious.
PRENATAL SUGGESTIONS	Not suitable.
HAVING TROUBLE?	My knees hurt when I come up.
TRY . . .	*Increase the distance between your knees. If this doesn't work, try using a tie around the ankles to reduce the flexion of the joint.*

Camel Pose (*Ustrasana*)

You'll Need

A few blankets
Possibly a wall and a block

Here's How

Camel Pose is an excellent posture to try out your newfound engagement of the hyoid and the frontal support of your spine. Work slowly through the variations, progressing to the next only if you can do so without strain to your lower back.

Variation A

Sit in a kneeling position. Slowly come up off your heels, bringing your thighs upright and turning your feet under. Place your hands firmly on the top of your buttocks. As you breathe, slowly begin to reach up and out through the top of the head, gradually moving the back into an arc. Keep your chin resting on your chest so you can concentrate on getting the maximum extension through your thoracic spine rather than extending through your neck alone. Each time you breathe in, expand the chest, opening the heart and lungs outward. As you breathe out, maintain the lift of the chest and move a little more into the arc. Press down into your knees and thighs to anchor your legs. This anchor will give you a platform from which to reach out through your spine (Figure 188). You have two options as to how to come out of the posture. You can rock toward your hips and then kneel (harder on your back but easier on your knees) or you can lower your buttocks into the kneeling position (harder on the knees but easier on your back). Do not twist as you come out by bringing one arm down and then the other, as this can seriously injure your back.

If you felt comfortable in the previous variation, now proceed to Variation B.

Variation B

Kneel with your back to a wall. Assume the first variation, except this time come farther back so that the back of your head is resting gently on the wall. Although this looks awkward, the wall allows you to relax your neck muscles so you can concentrate on opening the chest further. Now bring your hands to rest on your heels. If this is too much for your back, try raising your hands up onto blocks to reduce the angle in your back (Figure 189). Press down through your thighs and expand your spine up and out of the pelvis. Stay for three to five breaths and then release.

Final Position

If you've found the previous variations comfortable in your lower back, now complete the posture by bringing your hands all the way down onto the soles of your feet. If you are able to establish an almost horizontal position with your chest, you are now ready to allow the head to extend back (Figure 190). Don't be in a hurry to bring the head back until you've established enough opening in your thoracic spine to act as a foundation for your neck. As you stay, imagine increasing the negative space of the pose; that is, the space inside the posture should become bigger. Stay for several breaths, and then slowly release.

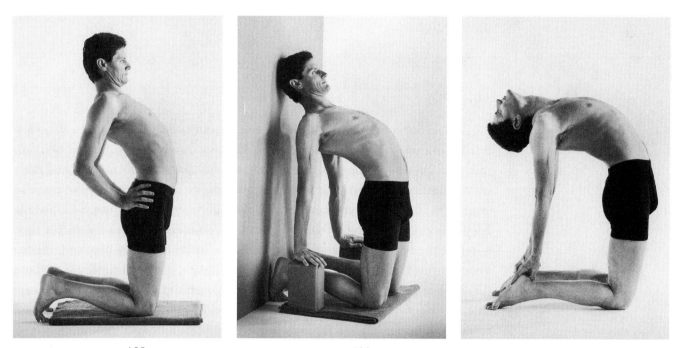

FIGURE 188   FIGURE 189   FIGURE 190

BENEFITS AND EFFECTS	Opens the groin, thighs, and entire back. Expands the chest, heart, and lungs. Releases excessive heat from the internal organs, especially the liver.
WHO SHOULDN'T DO THIS POSE	Those with spondylolisthesis or spondylolysis should practice the Camel only with the assistance of an experienced teacher. Those with arthritis or degeneration in the cervical spine should avoid bringing the head back if this causes a feeling of dizziness.
PRENATAL SUGGESTIONS	
HAVING TROUBLE?	I feel compression in my lower back even in the first variation.
TRY . . .	*You may have a very tight groin and/or upper back and shoulders that are causing you to seesaw on your lumbar spine. Try working with the Warrior Lunge and the Reclining Hero variations with one leg forward. Also work with the preparatory upper-back openers. Do these movements regularly and try the Camel occasionally to test for improvement.*

Cobra Pose (*Bhujangasana* I)

You'll Need

Several blankets

Here's How

Lie facedown with a folded blanket under your belly. Bring your hands to rest just behind your shoulders on the floor. As you exhale, draw your front body up into your back body, engaging the support of your hyoid to lift the head and chest off the floor. Lead from your chest, keeping the head in a neutral position. Use your arms to assist rather than dictate how high up you come. Unlike Upward-Facing Dog, the hips stay on the floor in Cobra Pose, and thus this is a deeper back bend. In the beginning it is advisable to keep your arms slightly bent and to keep your eyes level with the horizon or lower (Figure 191). This will allow you to focus on elongating your back and engaging the whole back in the action. When you are able to bring the chest into a vertical position while straightening the arms, you are ready to allow the head to arc back in a gesture of surrender (Figure 192). As you bring the head back, reach strongly back through your tail to elongate the back.

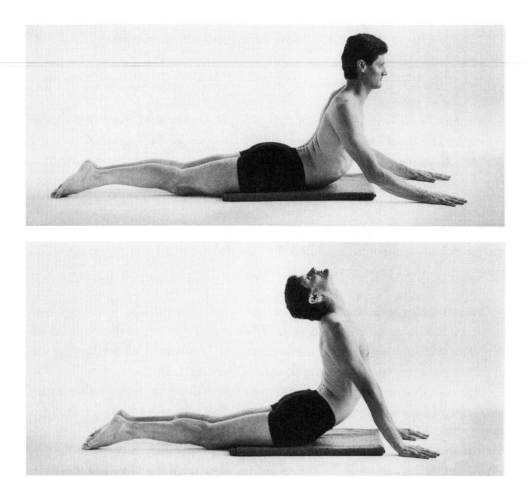

FIGURE 191

FIGURE 192

Stay for a few breaths before rolling down to rest on the floor. Take Child's Pose or Downward-Facing Dog to release your back.

BENEFITS AND EFFECTS	Strengthens and opens the entire back. Invigorates the heart and lungs and stimulates the sex, thymus, and thyroid glands. Reduces gas in the intestines and releases excessive heat trapped in the organs.
WHO SHOULDN'T DO THIS POSE	Those with spondylolisthesis or spondylolysis should practice the Cobra only with the assistance of an experienced teacher.
PRENATAL SUGGESTIONS	Only if comfortable.
HAVING TROUBLE?	I feel pressure in my lower back.
TRY ...	*Work with Upward-Facing Dog with your hands on blocks (page 119) to decrease the angle in your lower back. When this posture is comfortable, try Cobra again.*

Upward-Facing Bow (*Urdhva Dhanurasana*)

You'll Need

A folding chair and the help of two partners (if you want to try the assisted variation). Those with stiff wrists should use a wrist wedge (see page 28).

Here's How

Upward-Facing Bow is a dynamic back bend that requires a comprehensive preparation of shoulder-opening postures, movements to release the quadriceps and hip flexor muscles into extension, and simple back bends to prepare the whole spine (e.g., ball and chair work, Locust Pose, etc.).

Variation A (with chair)

In this first variation you'll use a chair to raise your feet higher than your shoulders. This will radically decrease the angle in your lower back while allowing you to focus your attention on opening your belly, chest, and shoulders.

Place a chair securely on top of your yoga mat with the back of the chair facing a wall. Lie down with your buttocks facing the chair and with your feet on the seat of the chair. Move close enough to the chair so that you can hold the chair legs with both hands. The important lesson in this preparation is that the basis of Upward Bow does not come solely from the strength of the arms and shoulders but is equally supported by the legs and the pelvis. On an exhalation press down through your feet and lift the hips off the floor in a fluid rolling motion. Extend your arms strongly downward as you lift through the core of your body. Rotate your hips inward to prevent your legs from falling outward and causing compression in the lumbar and sacral areas (Figure 193).

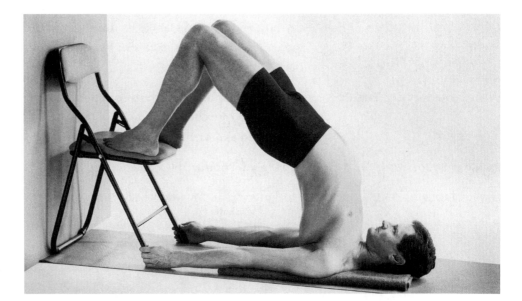

FIGURE 193

Variation B (with chair)

From the previous position now place your hands either side of your head with your fingers facing your shoulders. On an exhalation initiate the lift from your navel center, pressing through your legs and arms to lift your head and chest up off the floor. Lightly rest on the top of your head for a moment and then, on an exhalation, press strongly through your arms to come completely off the floor (Figure 194). To make this pose easier on your spine, come up onto your toes and open your chest away from the floor, keeping your head in a neutral position or pressing the chin to your chest to lift your sternum. Only when you can bring your chest into a vertical position with your arms completely straight should you attempt to let your head release backward. If you find that the tightness in your wrists prevents you from fully extending your arms, try elevating the base of your wrists with a wrist wedge (page 28). To come down, draw your head in toward your chest and slowly lower your buttocks to the floor. Rest completely. Repeat this variation several times.

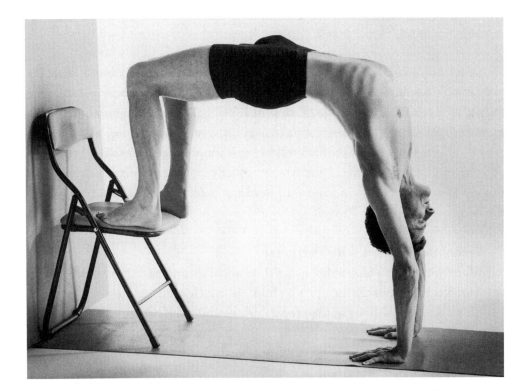

FIGURE 194

Final Position

Lie on your back with your knees bent and raise one foot at a time, letting your foot return to the ground where it falls naturally. This gives you an ideal placement for the heel-to-buttock distance. Take a moment to check that your feet have not turned out excessively. Place your palms on the floor with the tip of your middle finger in alignment with the middle of your shoulder joint. The elbows will be vertical.

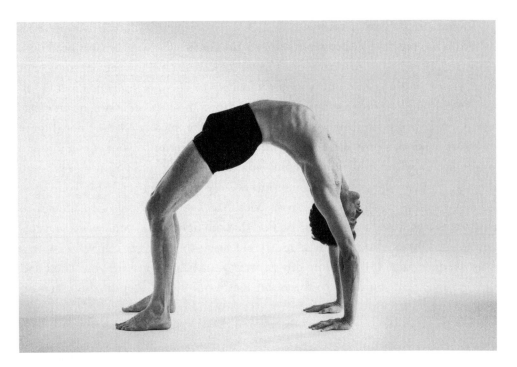

FIGURE 195

Shift your mental focus and breathe into the area just beneath the navel. In your mind's eye recapture the rolling movement of your spine that you developed during the preparations with the chair. When you make the commitment to move, there is a split second between the movement of your pelvis and legs and then the action of your arms and shoulders, following through to complete the lift. Open your abdomen and balance your weight equally between your hands and feet (Figure 195). To come down, raise your head and chin and slowly lower yourself to the floor.

Variation (Assisted with Partners)

When you first try Upward Bow on the floor, it's wonderful to have the help of two partners to encourage the opening from the navel center and the elongation in your back. Lie on the floor in the preparatory position and have your partners face you—one at your head, one at your feet. Place a yoga tie at the top of your buttocks (*not* your waist or in the crease of your lower back) and another tie just beneath the line of your armpits across the upper back and shoulder blades. Your partners will assist you by drawing the ties outward and slightly upward to stretch your back from head to tail. As they are carrying much of your body weight, their help will make it much easier if you have weak arms. On an exhalation come up, giving your partners feedback as to whether you need more or less support or if you need them to raise or lower the position of the ties. Use their assistance to elongate your back, attempting to bring your arms and chest into a vertical position. If you have very tight wrists, you can take hold of your helper's ankles. This will allow you to straighten your arms while the wrist is in a neutral position (Figure 196). Stay for several breaths before releasing to come down.

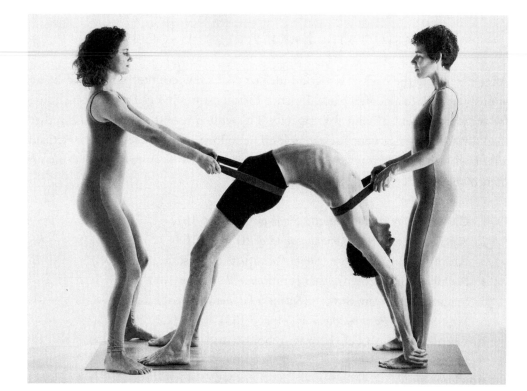

FIGURE 196

BENEFITS AND EFFECTS	Strengthens the shoulders, back, and legs. Invigorates the lungs, while releasing excess heat from the internal organs. Strongly stimulates the kidneys. Increases stamina.
WHO SHOULDN'T DO THIS POSE	Those with spondylolisthesis or spondylolysis should practice Upward Bow only with the assistance of an experienced teacher. Those with high blood pressure, detached retina, or glaucoma. Those with carpel tunnel syndrome in the wrists.
PRENATAL SUGGESTIONS	🔆, only if comfortable. The strong pull on the rectus abdominus muscles makes this unsuitable for later pregnancy.
HAVING TROUBLE?	My shoulders feel really locked.
TRY . . .	*Repetitions of the Sun Salutation will help to warm and loosen the shoulder joints. The Handstand and Elbow Stand as well as their preparatory postures will further liberate your shoulders. Shoulder Stretch Through the Chair (Variation B), Back Bend over Bolster, and Shoulder Chair Stretch are specific variations you should work on regularly.*

RELEASING THE BACK AFTER BACK BENDS

After extending the back it is a good idea to take a few counterpostures to bring your spine back to a neutral place. Practice these postures in brief repetitions, going for only 75 percent of your full capacity. This will ensure that you release rather than further challenge your back muscles. The following sequence can be practiced after back bends or, if you are short on time, one or two postures can be done on their own.

1. Crossed-Legs Twist (*Parivrtta Siddhasana*) (page 161)
2. Sage Pose I and II (*Bharadrajasana* I & II) (page 164)
3. Reclining Big-Toe Pose (*Supta Padangusthasana*) series (page 138)
4. Revolved Belly Pose (*Jathara Parivartanasana*) (page 162)
5. Supported Forward Stretch (*Salamba Uttanasana*) (page 114)
6. West Stretch (*Paschimottanasana*) (page 155)
7. Corpse Pose with a chair, or with bolster under the knees (*Savasana*) (page 239)

VI

Arm Balances and
Upside-Down Poses

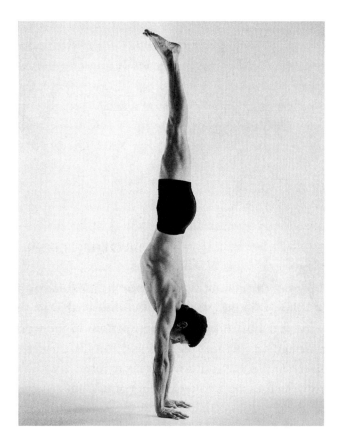

INTRODUCTION

*F*rom the core of the body our arms extend as projections of our heart and lungs. These physical extensions enable us to make manifest our inner dreams and aspirations as concrete actions in the world. When our arms become strong and can support the body, we can lift, carry, reach for, refuse, and remodel objects around us, making it possible to interact with the natural world on our own terms. Such strength fosters a sense of self-sufficiency—a natural ebullience that is marked in people such as carpenters and farmers, whose work is physically demanding.

The arm balances increase strength, flexibility, and range of motion throughout the shoulder girdle, which is essential for good alignment in the inversions. The inclusion of even a few arm balances within a daily practice rapidly warms the body and gradually builds stamina. For the average city dweller whose greatest demand may be carrying a bag of groceries once or twice a week, these postures can at first be quite challenging. Yet even after a month of their practice one can feel and *see* amazing changes in the musculature of the upper chest, shoulders, and arms. When there is inadequate upper-body strength, there is a tendency to transfer stress into the neck, making it vulnerable to injury. Fortifying the limbs, especially for women with delicate frames, can radically reduce neck problems.

The benefits of practicing such inversions as Headstand and Shoulder Stand can be viewed through two lenses. The Western perspective recognizes that these postures improve the circulation, nourish the endocrine glands, and promote a balance of all metabolic functions in the body. The unusual action of turning the body upside down stimulates the nervous system, increasing mental alertness and clarity. The Eastern perspective and justification for this strange reversal is quite different. *Asanas* such as Headstand were originally classified as *mudras,*[1] or sacred gestures, and were intended to have a far more dynamic action than the *asanas* and to effect deeper changes in the human personality. Unlike *asanas,* which the scriptures readily explicate, the ancient yogic texts treat *mudras* as highly secret techniques, enjoining the student to keep them concealed from the uninitiated. Yogis believed that the pineal gland in the head—which they viewed as a cooling, or "lunar" agent—secreted a special fluid of immortality called *amrita,* which in upright postures would drip down and be burned away by the solar plexus. By turning the body upside down, the *amrita* might be retained as a regenerative elixir, creating vibrant, glowing health. While this may seem far-fetched, there is an undeniable youthful glow that emanates from those who practice these poses regularly. When you practice the inversions consistently, they undoubtedly create an overall feeling of being "internally well groomed," with the accompanying feelings of freshness that one might experience briefly after a good haircut!

But health and longevity—obsessed as we are with these qualities today—were not the primary focus or concern of the ancient yogis. The fundamental intention of all yoga practices was to purify and calibrate the human system so that one might experience life at a higher resolution. Almost all such ancient technologies for this transformation focus on the upward movement of the raw, powerful energy in the lower chakras through all the other chakras to the crown of the head. The secret channel through which this energy flows is called the "hollow bamboo" by the Taoists, the "inner flute" by some Tantric texts, and the *Sushumna* by the yogis.[2] It begins at the perineum—the point that lies between the anus and the genitals— and moves up through the body to the crown of the head.

This energetic pathway is not generally recognized as an anatomical reality by Western science. However the channel does follow through the body actual physical and neurological pathways that connect the endocrine glands. In effect, the inversions "irrigate" these subtle pathways, stimulating their latent potential. By opening and vitalizing this channel, a practitioner may be able to experience a concomitant refinement of consciousness that will allow access to deeper and more subtle layers of the body and mind.

INVERSIONS AND MENSTRUATION

During menstruation avoid turning the body upside down. When the body is inverted, gravity causes the vessels supplying blood to the uterus to be partially blocked, and this can temporarily stop the flow.[3] From the Eastern viewpoint the energy of the body at this time in a woman's cycle is moving down into the earth.

Going upside down during the menses disturbs this natural rhythm and can result in a feeling of shakiness and disorientation. Additionally, arm balances that strongly contract the abdomen feel harsh at this time of the month. Honor your body during your moon cycle by going *with* rather than *against* this natural flow.

KEY MOVING PRINCIPLES FOR THE ARM BALANCES AND UPSIDE-DOWN POSES

4. CENTER

Maintain the Integrity of the Spine: The Central Axis

5. SUPPORT

Establish Foundations of Support: Structural Building Blocks

6. ALIGN

Create Clear Lines of Force: Alignment and Sequential Flow

7. ENGAGE

Engage the Whole Body: Review the Glands

ESSENTIAL SKILLS

The Hands: Foundations of Support

~ Distributing Weight Through the Hands

Unlike our predecessors who walked on all fours, what defines us as human is our preference for standing on our feet, thus liberating our hands for other uses. When we once again stand on our hands, as we do in so many of the postures that follow, the hands become equal to the feet as bases of support, giving rise to a sense of primal connection to our early roots as quadruped animals.

Where you put the weight through your hands has a powerful cascade effect into the wrist, elbow, shoulder, and neck. Take a look at your upturned left palm now. Notice that there is a slight hollow in the center of the palm, much like the arch of the foot. From this hollow the palm rises into mounds like gentle hills that surround a valley. Use your right index finger to trace a pathway around this handscape. Start in the center of the palm and then glide the index finger toward the base of the thumb. Now make a slow circle around the perimeter of the palm, noticing that there is a slight depression between the pad of the thumb and the pads at the base of the fingers, and that there is also a depression at the center of the wrist between the outer and inner wrist. When you place your hands on the floor as the base of support for a posture, the weight should be predominantly on the fleshy mounds of the palm and equally distributed throughout the length of the fingers (Figure 198). It's especially important that you do not collapse at the depression at the center of the wrist. The median nerve passes through this depression, and collapsing weight through this part of the wrist or hyperextending the wrist can damage this nerve, causing serious problems such as carpal tunnel syndrome.

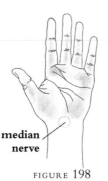

median nerve

FIGURE 198

People often experience strain in the wrists when practicing arm balances, which is why many students exclude them from their practice altogether. Some of this strain is due to a lack of conditioning in the muscles of the forearm, but most difficulties in this area can be avoided by observing the following precautions:

～ Never practice arm balances of any kind on a soft, yielding surface, such as carpet or sand, where the base of the wrist drops below the level of the fingers. This hyperextends and damages the wrist. A nonslip mat placed on top of a hardwood or linoleum floor is ideal.

～ Place the hands so the creases of the wrists are horizontal to the wall in front of you. This will ensure that even pressure is being placed on both the inner and outer wrist. It will also ensure that your elbows and shoulders are turning neither in nor out.

～ Spread your fingers as wide as possible from the thumb to the little finger so the palm is very broad. This placement will distribute the weight over a greater surface area, reducing strain on any one part of the wrist.

～ If you feel strain in the wrists, try lifting the base of the wrist with a wrist wedge or slant board (page 28) to reduce the angle of extension.

～ Condition the body slowly by including a few weight-bearing poses in every practice session, rather than straining yourself by doing arm balances once a month.

～ INQUIRY ～

The Arms Mirror the Hands

Take a simple posture like Downward-Facing Dog for which you are on all fours. Before you come into the posture, spread the hands wide from thumbs across to the little fingers, and align the wrists so that there is equal pressure on the inner and outer base of the palms. Maintain this equal distribution of weight as you come up into the posture.

Now deliberately shift your weight to different parts of your hands. Let your weight rock onto the outside of the hands, allowing the inner wrists and thumbs to lift. Notice that as you do this the outer wrists compress, and the muscles along the outer edges of your arms and shoulders are doing all the work. Now let the weight drop into the base of the wrists. Notice that as you do this the undersides of the arms and shoulders open while the tops of the arms and shoulders close. Now shift the weight forward to the base of the fingers, lifting the base of the wrists as you do so. Notice that this activates the muscles along the tops of the arms and opens the shoulder joints. Now let the weight shift to the inside of your hands. Observe how the inner muscles of your arms and shoulders engage. In essence, how you place the weight through your hands has a direct effect on how you use your arms. Now distribute the weight evenly again. To reduce strain at the base of the wrists, focus on lifting the forearms away from the floor so the weight of your body is carried by the front of your hands and fingers. Find the position where your arms and shoulders feel as if they are working equally engaged—upper, lower, inner, and outer working in synchrony. Can you identify the effects this equal or unequal distribution of weight has had on other areas of your body?

THE HEAD AS CENTRAL SUPPORT

You may have admired the grace of native peoples carrying provisions balanced on their heads. These people intuitively understand that the least stressful position for carrying added weight is neither in front, behind, nor to the side of the body, but directly over the central axis. By elongating the spine upward against the weight above the head, such people maintain the spaces between the vertebrae of the neck and develop strong, steady musculature to support the span between the bones.

We need to create a similar dynamic in the head and neck when the head is used as the base of support in postures such as Headstand. To simulate the correct feeling in your head and neck, find a large, heavy book or object that can be easily balanced. Place it directly on top of your head. Elongate up through the crown of your head as you descend down through your heels. Notice that if you lift your chin, the book will fall. Spend a few minutes walking and standing, then remove the weight. Can you feel a new lightness and ease in your neck and head? This is the sensation you want to re-create in Headstand.

FRAMING THE HEAD

One common misconception about Headstand is that the weight of the body should pass through the arms, not the head. While it is true that beginners should first learn to carry most of the weight with the arms, so they can modulate the amount of weight coming through the neck when alignment is still crude, this technique is a means to an end, and not the end itself. When you learn how to use the arms correctly and to draw the shoulders away from the ears, the shoulder girdle and arms will create a frame that enables the neck successfully to elongate and bear weight.

Problems occur in Headstand when the shoulders collapse down or out, destroying the "frame." When the inner architecture of the frame is faulty, the muscles collapse or move in the wrong direction, and the spaces between the cervical vertebrae narrow. The cervical curve may become flattened or accentuated. This distortion makes it impossible for your bones to carry the weight of your body effectively.

～ INQUIRY ～

The Frame of the Head, Neck, and Shoulders

An excellent pose for learning how to create this frame for the neck is Expanded-Leg Pose (page 111). Stand with your feet very wide apart and your toes turned slightly in. Pivot forward from your hips and place your hands on the floor, shoulder-width apart, with your fingertips in line with the toes. Spread your fingers wide, and bend the elbows so your forearms form a right angle to the floor. Broaden your shoulders away from your spine and roll them back away from your ears. Extend your elbows away from your face and draw them in so the tips of your elbows align to your hands. With the frame you have created from the heads of your shoulders across your shoulder blades and down through the arms, your neck will now be able to elongate toward the floor (Figure 199).

The more common tendency, however, is to let the shoulders round toward the

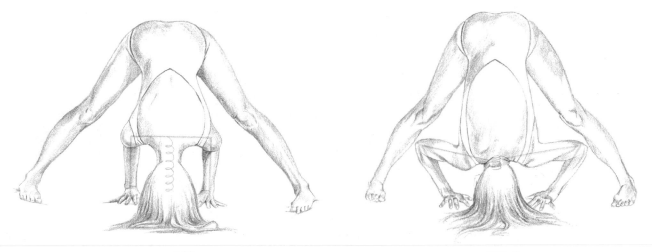

FIGURE 199   FIGURE 200. *Incorrect*

ears and the arms splay outward. This collapsed frame causes the neck to compress and be unable to bear weight effectively (Figure 200). When you have a clear sense of the correct position of the neck, head, and arms in a non-weight-bearing position, you are ready to proceed to Headstand.

USING THE WALL FOR SUPPORT

In many of the postures that follow, you will be learning to balance upside down. This requires a new neuromuscular coordination that at first will be quite perplexing. The exhilaration of balancing for even a second in mid-space, however, will make the practice and effort required seem a meager investment. In this nascent stage it's helpful and safer to work with the support of the wall. How you use the wall, however, will determine whether it is aiding you in learning how to balance or creating a permanent crutch that will hinder your progress.

Guidelines

1. Correct Distance from the Wall. Place your hands, head, or elbows (depending on the posture) one shin-length away from the wall. Because everyone's body proportions are different, you'll need to measure this. Sit on the floor facing the wall, with your legs straight in front of you and your feet against the wall. The distance from your feet to your knees is one shin-length. Your base of support should be positioned where your knees are on the floor. Eventually you'll be able to eyeball the distance. Here's the reason for this careful measuring.

2. Use the Wall Actively, *Not* Passively. As you come up into an inversion, place both feet against the wall and bend the knees so your shins are perpendicular to the wall. Later when you become more adept, you can just touch the wall with one foot. This positioning will allow you to use your abdominal, pelvic floor, and hamstring muscles to bring the pelvis into an upright position. When you feel the pelvis coming over the trunk with the tail actively lifted, you can try extending one leg straight above you. (Figure 201a). Draw the pubic bone toward the navel to connect the legs to the abdomen. Once your have this balance you can then tentatively take the second leg off the wall for a freestanding balance. Using the wall this way, you are teaching the body what it must do to be able to go up into a freestanding balance without support.

In Figure 201b I have shown the more common and incorrect usage of the wall. Here the person is closer to the wall and is leaning the weight of the legs into the wall. You can see that if the wall were removed he would fall backward imme-

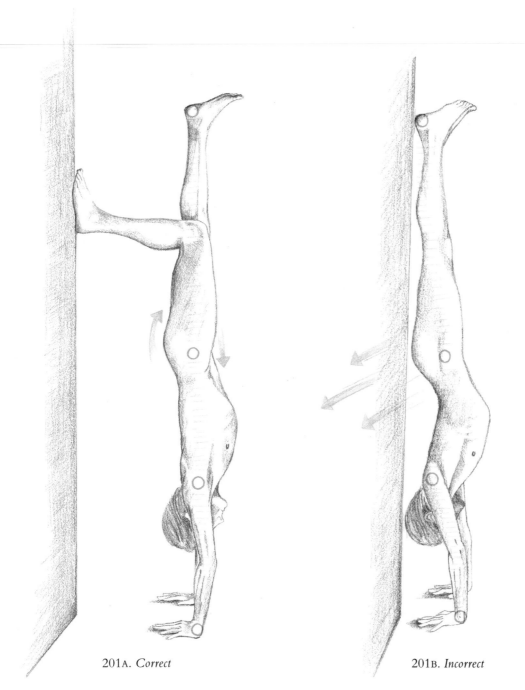

201A. *Correct*   201B. *Incorrect*

diately. Because both legs are straight and behind the line of the pelvis, the abdominal muscles are completely released, making it impossible to gain control over the core support of the limbs. Also the trunk is behind the vertical line of the arms, causing strain and a poor carrying angle through the arms. This person is teaching himself how to fall. If he tried to balance in the center of the room, he would catapult himself into a nifty back flip! While being closer to the wall gives a psychological sense of security, this position is not any safer and patterns the muscles to do exactly the opposite of what they need to do to balance.

THE ARM BALANCES AND UPSIDE-DOWN POSES

One-Arm Stand (*Vasisthasana*)

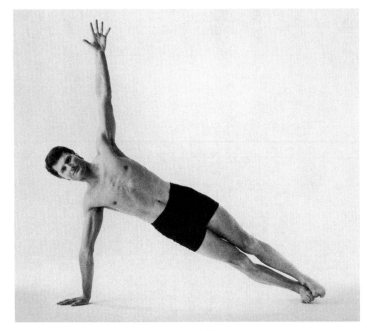

FIGURE 202

Here's How

Start in Downward-Facing Dog (page 116) and slowly revolve the whole body until you are balanced on the outside of your right foot and on the surface of the right hand. Align the center of your palm with the arch of the back foot so your body is in one line. Keeping the trunk stable, open your chest and slowly extend your left arm out from the chest. Breathe, filling the chest and extending all the limbs stridently from the core of the body (Figure 202). Stay for three full breaths, then return to Downward-Facing Dog and practice on the second side. This is a fun pose to include as a part of the Sun Salutation (page 125), where it can be practiced after Dog Pose or immediately after the first lunge when you bring the second leg back.

BENEFITS AND EFFECTS	Increases arm and abdominal strength. Improves flexibility of the wrists. Improves balance and stamina.
WHO SHOULDN'T DO THIS POSE	Those with carpal tunnel syndrome or occupational overuse syndrome.
PRENATAL SUGGESTIONS	
HAVING TROUBLE?	I can't seem to balance.
TRY . . .	*Try wedging your foot against a wall for support. You may also be collapsing your torso into the supporting arm. Make the chest buoyant so that the chest and arms form an open cross.*

East Stretch (*Purvottanasana*)

Here's How

Sit in Stick Pose (page 133) with your legs extended in front of you. Place your palms down on either side of your hips. Your fingers can either point toward your

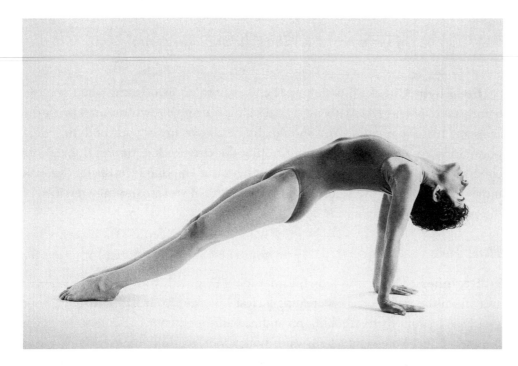

FIGURE 203

feet or away from your feet—each has a different effect on the shoulders. On an inhalation slowly bend the knees and lift the buttocks and trunk off the floor. Focus on lifting the tailbone up and under as you draw the pubic bone toward the navel to prevent the pelvis from overarching. Press strongly down through the arms, lifting the chest up, keeping the head and eyes looking down toward the chest. Do not arch your head backward until you can raise the chest to touch the chin. If your back is still comfortable, straighten the legs, pointing the toes and allowing the head to release back to complete this magnificent arch through the whole body (Figure 203). Take three full breathes and slowly lower yourself onto the floor. This pose can also be entered from the One-Arm Stand, by pivoting on the supporting hand and revolving over into the supported arch.

BENEFITS AND EFFECTS	Strengthens the arms and opens and clears the chest. Strengthens the legs and abdominal muscles. Releases tension in the shoulders.
WHO SHOULDN'T DO THIS POSE	Those with carpal tunnel syndrome or occupational overuse syndrome.
PRENATAL SUGGESTIONS	
HAVING TROUBLE?	My lower back hurts when I straighten my legs.
TRY . . .	*If tucking the tail under does not alleviate this, try flexing your feet instead of pointing your toes. If this does not alleviate the discomfort, raise the hands onto blocks and work with bent knees.*

Handstand (*Adho Mukha Vrksasana*)

Pre-Flight Check: You are physically ready to do Handstand when you can comfortably practice Downward-Facing Dog for one to two minutes with the arms and torso in one line. You should also be able to lower your body in Four-Limb Stick Pose (page 122) without resting the chest or legs on the floor. Build confidence and strength in these poses first before attempting Handstand. (Keep in mind that these objective yardsticks may mean little if you are mortally terrified of the very idea of turning upside down!)

Here's How

Beginners: Come into Downward-Facing Dog with your hands shin-length away from the wall. Focus on creating a clear line from your hands through your shoulders to your torso, reaching up and back through your tailbone to lengthen the back. Lunge your right leg forward about a foot, gently arching the neck as you look at the floor between the hands (Figure 204). Bending both knees, yield into the floor and spring your left leg and then your right up over your head. Keep your head up so that you are looking at the floor in front of your hands. As your feet touch the wall, carefully bend both knees and begin to draw your tailbone up by lifting through the back of the pelvis and contracting the abdomen. As you feel confident, extend one leg over your body (Figure 205). If you are steady here, take the second leg up over your body for the full balance (Figure 206). Breathe deeply as you concentrate on holding your balance. When you are ready to come down, bend both knees again, allowing the ankles, knees, and hips to release as you touch the floor. Rest in Forward Stretch (page 113) or Downward-Facing Dog before coming up to standing.

Advanced: Once you feel confident coming up at the wall one leg at a time, you are ready to try coming up with both legs together. Coming up with one leg at a time may seem easier, but this entry method tends to twist the pelvis and can torque the back if done repeatedly. In this more elegant ascent you begin in Downward-Facing Dog, but instead of stepping one foot forward, you slowly walk both legs in toward the head until the hips are balanced over the chest; then spring up with both legs together. As you walk the feet closer in toward

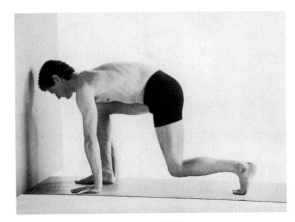

FIGURE 204

the body to bring the pelvis over the chest, you need to lift the spine in and up off the arms and reach strongly through the tail. Practice taking a few bunny-hop bounces with both legs bent. Make sure that you are releasing your knees and ankles, as this will allow you to create the momentum to spring up. When you are ready, bend the knees deeply and spring up, swinging the pelvis over your head with the thighs drawn in close to the abdomen (Figure 207). One common error in coming up with both legs is to kick the legs out away from the body or to splay the legs apart—this makes it impossible to control the legs, as they are too far away from the center of gravity. Just as you did before, go through the same steps using the wall as support and, when you are confident, take both legs away from the wall (Figure 206).

Once you are confidently practicing Handstand coming up with both legs at the wall, you are ready to practice the posture in the middle of the room. If you find this daunting, ask a fellow yoga buddy or your teacher to spot you from behind. If you are working alone, the best way to fall is to relax the arms slightly and let the legs fall behind the head onto the floor into a relaxed back bend. Some helpful hints: Much of your work in learning to balance will be in modulating the amount of force you need to get up. The degree of force you use to get up is the same force you will need to stop to balance. Experiment with how little force you can use and still get the legs in the air. Once your legs are over your head, contract the muscles at the base of your buttocks and thighs to draw the sitting bones toward the backs of the knees. This action will prevent your pelvis and legs from falling backward. Simultaneously, draw your pubic bone toward your navel so that your abdominal muscles are activated to hold your pelvis steady. Practice this

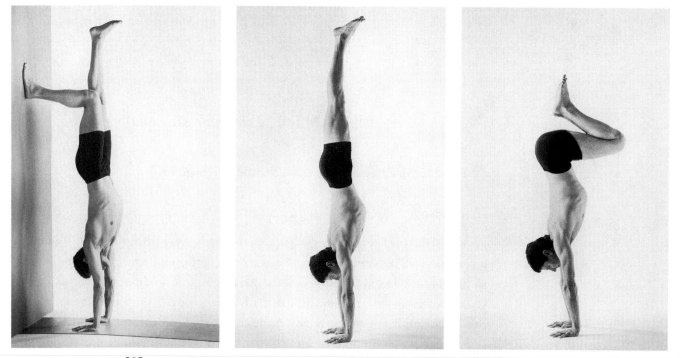

FIGURE 205   FIGURE 206   FIGURE 207

action while standing upright before trying it upside down. Getting the knack of this balance may take many months of practice, but the sheer exhilaration of balancing on the hands is worth every bit of the effort.

BENEFITS AND EFFECTS	Brings lightness and focus to the mind and body. Strengthens the arms, shoulder girdle, and abdominal muscles. Alleviates fatigue and sleepiness. Develops coordination, balance, and neuromuscular integration.
WHO SHOULDN'T DO THIS POSE	Those with carpal tunnel syndrome or any other wrist injury irritated by extreme extension. Those who have high blood pressure, detached retina, or glaucoma. Those with hyperextended elbows or injuries to the shoulder girdle should practice only with the help of an experienced teacher.
PRENATAL SUGGESTIONS	*if* you practiced this posture with ease before you became pregnant, and as long as it feels comfortable for you.
HAVING TROUBLE?	My legs don't seem to come off the ground!
TRY . . .	*For most people this is a fear issue and is best handled by having an experienced teacher stand behind you at the wall. When there is fear, the knees lock and prevent the body from coiling enough to get the momentum to come up. Placing two bolsters on the floor against the wall in front of your hands can create psychological security if you are working alone.*

Elbow Stand (*Pinchamayurasana*)

Pre-Flight Check: Same as for Handstand (page 216).

Here's How

Kneel facing a wall with the arms shin-length away from the wall. Place your forearms shoulders-width apart on a yoga mat, with the fingers strongly extended so the thumbs and index fingers form a right angle. Some people find using two yoga mats gives a more comfortable cushioning for the sensitive elbows. Check that your weight is being carried on the outer edge of the forearm and elbow—if you are resting on the inner edges of your elbows, your shoulders will turn inward and the elbows will splay apart when you come up. Now lift your hips up into

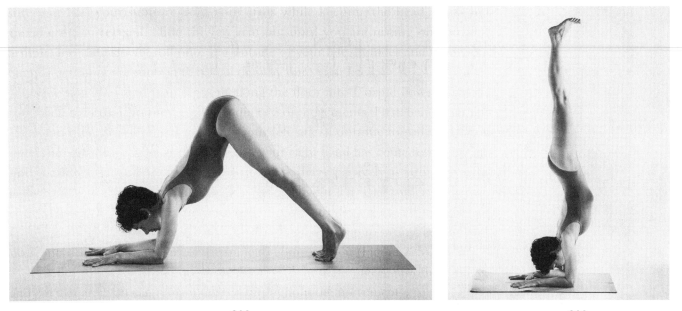

FIGURE 208   FIGURE 209

Downward-Facing Dog—it's exactly the same posture except that now you are supporting yourself on your forearms instead of your hands. Focus on lifting the pelvis up off the back and drawing the back in and up so there is space in the shoulder joints (Figure 208). Lift the head and arch the neck gently, looking at the space slightly in front of your hands. Carefully step one foot forward and, bending both knees, spring your legs up over your head one at a time. Go through the steps of using the wall for support just as you did for Handstand, graduating to the center of the room when you are comfortable at the wall.

When you do bring both legs up over the head, whether at the wall or in the center of the room, press the forearms strongly into the ground as you lift the chest off of the shoulders. Balance this action by reaching stridently up through your legs (Figure 209).

When you become confident of your balance in Elbow Stand, you can include it as a part of the Sun Salutation (page 125). When you take your Downward-Facing Dog, simply lower the elbows to the floor one at a time and alight into Elbow Stand. Balance and then return to Downward-Facing Dog before proceeding with the cycle.

BENEFITS AND EFFECTS	Warms and invigorates the entire body. Deeply releases the entire shoulder girdle. Strengthens the upper body.
WHO SHOULDN'T DO THIS POSE	Those with high blood pressure, detached retina, or glaucoma.
PRENATAL SUGGESTIONS	*if* you practiced this posture before you became pregnant, and only if it is comfortable.

HAVING TROUBLE?

As I try to come up I collapse onto my head.

TRY ...

This is a strength issue. Practice just the preparation with the elbows on the floor in Downward-Facing Dog for at least a month, until you can hold it for one minute. Do not attempt to come up until you can create a straight line from your arms through to your tail. Get a friend to check this for you.

Headstand (*Sirsasana*)

(A note on the sequencing of Headstand and Shoulder Stand: Referred to respectively as the king and queen of all the asanas, these two postures are energetically related. Headstand tends to heat the body and stimulate the nervous system and strongly tones the neck muscles. Shoulder Stand tends to cool or neutralize the body and sedates the nervous system while releasing the muscles of the neck and shoulders. In practice together, the logical sequence is to do Headstand first, followed by Shoulder Stand either immediately after, or later in your practice session. Headstand can leave you feeling very stimulated, so once it's done you really are committed to doing the other. Shoulder Stand can be safely practiced on its own as it has the amazing ability to neutralize the nervous system—if one comes to the practice agitated, it rapidly calms the body and mind; if one enters with flat batteries, it rapidly lifts and refreshes.)

Here's How

Place a folded blanket on top of your yoga mat shin-length away from the wall. Kneel in front of the blanket and loosely interlock your fingers, leaving the webbing between the last two little fingers slightly open. Place the hands and elbows on the floor, forming a tripod with the elbows shoulders-width apart. Look down

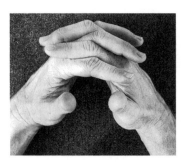

FIGURE 210

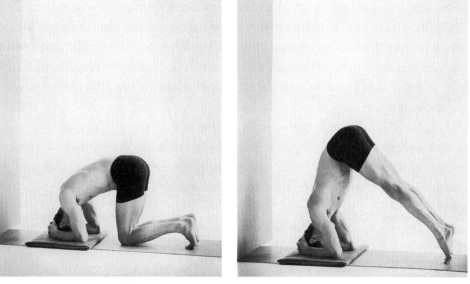

FIGURE 211

FIGURE 212

at your wrists. If you lift your thumbs upward, you will see a small indentation, called the "snuff box," on the top of the inner wrist. When your hands and arms are placed correctly, this little indentation should look directly upright, so that if it rained it would collect a drop of water (Figure 210). If the indentation turns downward, your shoulders are collapsing inward toward the neck, and the elbows have splayed outward. If the indentation falls outward, the outer shoulders will drop. Refer back to this indentation often to determine whether you have collapsed your frame for Headstand. Every time you practice Headstand, change the interlock of your hands (i.e., if you usually have your right index finger on top, interlace your fingers so the left is on top). This will ensure that you work both sides of the body evenly.

From a kneeling position, now bring your head onto your blanket, cupping the back of your head with your hands and placing your head with the weight slightly toward your forehead (Figure 211). Lift the pelvis off the floor, bringing your weight onto your arms and your head as you reach up and back with the pelvis in a modified Downward-Facing Dog. When you first learn this pose, use the arms to control the amount of weight you are releasing through the head and neck—try just letting your hair touch the floor, then the skin of the scalp, then the muscles of the scalp, then the skull, then the weight of the brain, testing at each stage that your neck is comfortable (Figure 212).

If you are new to the pose, come up by lightly springing one leg at a time and using the wall to help support you (Figure 213). Please review the "Essential Skills" section on how to use the wall safely and effectively. When you have become stronger and more flexible in your hips and shoulders, you can slowly walk your feet in toward your head to bring the pelvis over the chest. As you bring your legs closer to your head, be careful to lift your spine in and up and to draw your shoulders away from your ears and outward to create a strong frame for your neck.

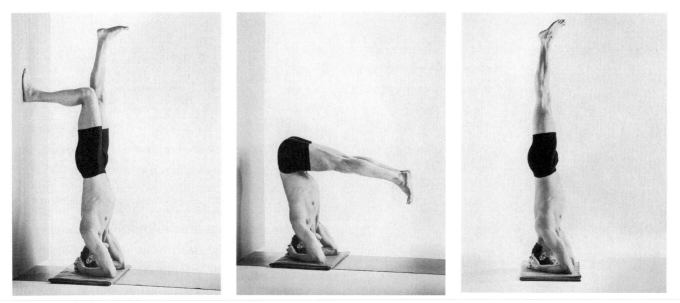

FIGURE 213   FIGURE 214   FIGURE 215

Depending on your flexibility, you can either hop up lightly with both legs together and with your knees bent, or slowly raise both straightened legs (Figure 214) into the full pose (Figure 215).

While in Headstand, experiment with where your weight is comfortably received through your head and neck—some people need to bring the weight more toward the forehead, while others feel best directly over the crown. Once you have established a strong frame with your arms and shoulders and the neck is elongating, you can allow more and more weight to come through your head. Counter this yielding action of the head by reaching strongly up through the perineum and through your inner thighs, inner calves, and the base of the big toes. Lifting from these inner muscles will help draw the body up along the central axis. Stay for one minute, gradually building up your stay in this posture, thirty seconds per month. This may sound conservative, but the neck and nervous system need to be conditioned slowly, and by gradually increasing your stay in the pose (up to ten minutes), you can back off if you experience a reaction to it.

To come down, slowly lower your legs—either straight or with bent knees—keeping your weight toward your forehead and elbows as you come down, so as not to collapse into your neck. Rest with your head on the floor in Child's Pose (page 193) for a good minute before sitting up.

BENEFITS AND EFFECTS	Stimulates the nervous system, increasing mental alertness and clarity. Nourishes and balances the endocrine system and all metabolic functions. Increases and improves circulation and prevents the buildup of fluid in the legs. Heats the body and increases gastric fire—prolonged practice may contribute to weight regulation. Together with Shoulder Stand, helps promote bowel regularity.
WHO SHOULDN'T DO THIS POSE	Those with high blood pressure, detached retina, glaucoma, or hiatal hernia. Those with neck injuries that would be exacerbated by increased weight through the cervical vertebrae. Do not practice if you are menstruating.
PRENATAL SUGGESTIONS	*If you practiced this pose before you became pregnant, and only if it is comfortable.*
HAVING TROUBLE?	My neck hurts *after* I come out of Headstand.
TRY . . .	*Like many people, you may have undiagnosed pre-existing weaknesses in your neck. Most common of these is simply a flattening of the normal cervical curve. Do not experiment on your own with this pose—seek the help of an experienced yoga teacher.*

Shoulder Stand (*Salamba Sarvangasana*)

You'll Need

4 blankets
A yoga mat
Possibly a tie and a second mat

Here's How

If you are new to Shoulder Stand, the safest way to enter this posture is with the support of a wall. Place a neatly folded stack of three to four blankets about 6 inches from the wall, with the folded edges facing away from the wall. Place a yoga mat under and over the blankets, leaving a 4-inch gap over the outer folded edge. The yoga mat is there to prevent the blankets from moving and to prevent your elbows from sliding apart—it should not be under your neck, head, and hair or it will prevent you from releasing these areas out away from your shoulders. The purpose of elevating your shoulders on the blankets is to reduce the degree of flexion through your neck. In a well-supported posture the teacher should be able to lift your head slightly off the floor. This little test means that your neck ligaments still have a little "give." When the posture is practiced on the floor without support, most people will be at 100 percent of their flexion and ligamental stretch (the head cannot be lifted), which leaves little room for error and increases the likelihood of strain. Experiment with the number of blankets you need to feel comfortable. Some people feel better with only two, while others need as many as six to practice comfortably.

Recline on the blankets with your shoulders about 3 inches from the folded edge and your head on the floor. Your buttocks should almost touch the wall when your shoulders are on the blankets, so if necessary roll over and adjust the distance before you continue. Place your feet on the wall and slowly begin to lift your pelvis and spine off the floor, leading with the tail, until your weight is over your shoulders. Interlock your hands behind your back and stretch the arms toward the wall to open the shoulders. As you do so, "walk" onto the top of your shoulders (Figure 216). Draw your arms inward so they are no wider than your shoulders. If your arms have a tendency to splay wide apart, which is common when the shoulders are very stiff, tie a yoga belt around your upper arms just above the elbow, cinching it in to the width of your shoulders.

Now place your hands on your back with your fingers reaching up the back toward your buttocks. It's best to have your hands right on your skin so you can lift the upper back in and up, working the hands as close to the neck as possible. As the chest comes upright allow your heels to come away from the wall (Figure 217). If your back is still very rounded or your elbows are coming off the floor, do not proceed past this point.

At this stage you should stay for about a minute to see how your neck is responding to the challenge of the posture. If your neck is at all uncomfortable, you should come down. An excellent way to reduce the degree of flexion in the neck for those whose upper backs and shoulders are so tight that the elbows lift off the mat is to use a stack of five blankets and place a tightly rolled mat under the elbows. You can further adjust the angle through the neck by placing one or two blankets directly under the head and neck (Figure 218).

If you are comfortable in the previous positions, now you are ready to take the feet off the wall. Extend one leg up in the air and begin to draw the tailbone in toward the pubic bone to tone the pelvic floor and to prevent your pelvis from tipping backward. Also contract the muscles at the base of your thighs and buttocks to lift the back of the pelvis up, simultaneously drawing the abdominal muscles inward. Now extend your second leg, reaching strongly upward through the inner edges of the leg and through the bases of your big toes, balls of your feet, and your heels (Figure 219). If this is your first time in Shoulder Stand, stay for one minute, gradually increasing your stay over a period of weeks and months until you can stay for ten minutes. To come down, bend your knees and touch your feet to the wall and slowly round your back into your hands, supporting yourself as you lower your back onto the blankets. Once down, shift your body until your head and shoulders

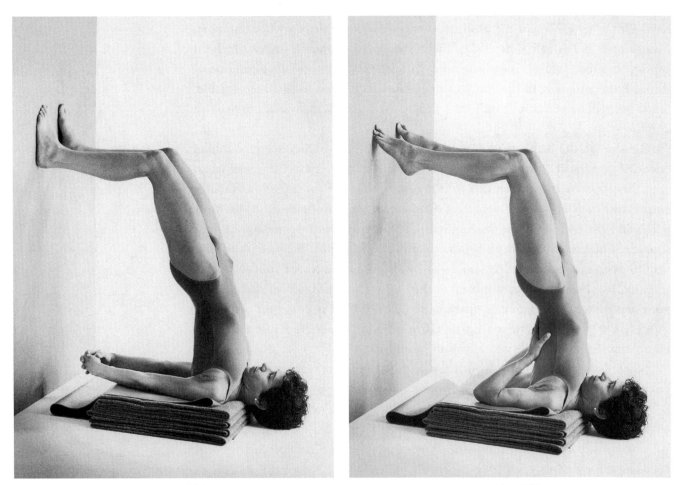

FIGURE 216   FIGURE 217

are *off* the edge of the blanket and your buttocks and lower back are supported on the blanket. Rest here for a few moments before you roll onto your side. Stay here at least a minute, letting your blood pressure adjust before sitting up.

Advanced: A wonderful sequence for entering Shoulder Stand freestanding is to begin by taking a relaxed Knee-to-Ear Pose (page 228) with your knees above your head on either side of your ears and with your weight resting on the *back* of the shoulders. Breathe deeply into your back, staying here for a minute or more until you can feel the back muscles lengthening and the area around the kidneys releasing. Now interlock your hands behind your back and extend your arms, releasing your shoulders back and under as you straighten your legs and lift the tail up into Plow Pose (page 226). Replace your hands on your back to lift the spine in and up, and stay here for a minute or more, lifting strongly up through the backs of the thighs to elongate the spine. Then come up into Shoulder Stand one leg at a time. If you are a more advanced student, you can complete this cycle by taking one or more of the Shoulder Stand variations (See *Light on Yoga*, by B. K. S. Iyengar, for instructions for the variations) and then returning for one last long, deep Knee-to-Ear Pose before entering relaxation.

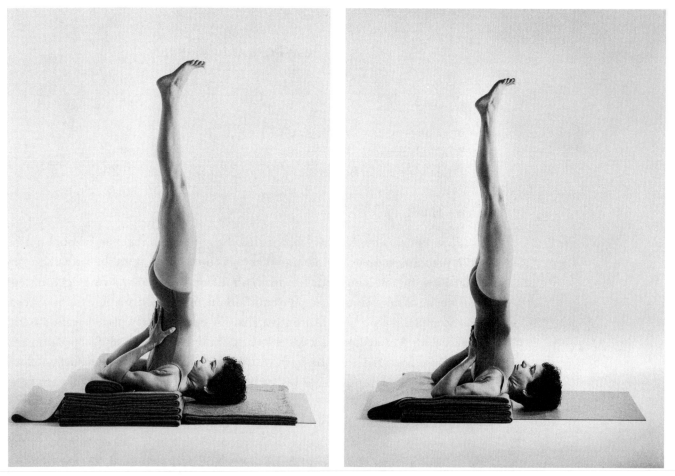

FIGURE 218   FIGURE 219

BENEFITS AND EFFECTS
Stimulates the balanced function of the endocrine glands and all metabolic functions. Sedates and neutralizes the nervous system, producing a profound sense of calm and ease. Improves circulation and reduces edema in the legs, feet, and ankles as well as reducing general fluid retention. Tones the internal organs (especially the uterus), and promotes bowel regularity.

WHO SHOULDN'T DO THIS POSE
Those with high blood pressure, detached retina, glaucoma, or hiatal hernia. Those with injuries to the neck that would be exacerbated by increased weight through the cervical vertebrae. Do not practice if you are menstruating.

PRENATAL SUGGESTIONS
(as long as it is comfortable).

HAVING TROUBLE?
I feel discomfort in my neck during and after this posture.

TRY ...
Because this is a complex posture, seek the help of an experienced teacher.

Plow Pose (*Halasana*)

You'll Need

Yoga mat
3 or 4 blankets
Possibly a chair or bolster

Here's How

Plow Pose is slightly more challenging than Shoulder Stand and should not be attempted unless one is already familiar and comfortable with the latter. You can enter Plow by lowering your legs from Shoulder Stand or by swinging your legs over the head from your starting position on the mat. If you are new to Plow Pose, I recommend raising your feet onto a chair or bolster, safely placed against a wall (Figure 220). This will make it easier to bring your back into a vertical position and will reduce potential strain on both your back and neck. You can gradually reduce the support by then practicing with a bolster, then a block, and finally with your feet on the floor.

To enter the posture from a reclining position, begin as you did for Shoulder Stand, working now in the center of the room. With a little rocking motion, round the back and swing your legs with the knees bent over your head. Keep your knees bent for a few moments, giving the back a chance to release. Then interlock your

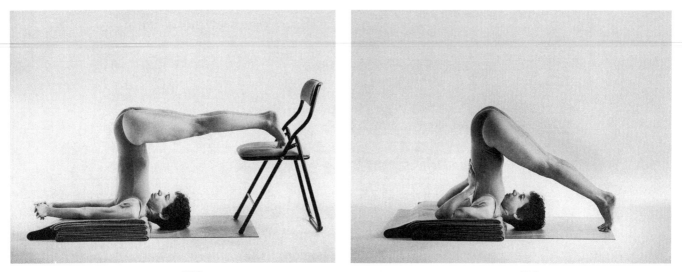

FIGURE 220   FIGURE 221

fingers and extend your arms behind your back as you lift your pelvis and spine upward, straightening your legs as you do so. Adjust the distance of the feet to the body until the back forms a right angle to the floor. Now replace the hands onto your back (on your skin is better than on top of your clothes) and lift your chest in and up (Figure 221). Stay for one to three minutes, breathing deeply into the back as you stay. You can either now come up into Shoulder Stand or proceed on to Knee-to-Ear Pose (page 228), *or* slowly roll down through your back until you are resting in Corpse Pose. It's a good idea to bend your knees and roll them to the left and to the right a few times to release the back muscles before entering relaxation.

BENEFITS AND EFFECTS	Stimulates the endocrine system, balancing metabolic function. Tones and releases tension in the abdominal organs. Strengthens the back.
WHO SHOULDN'T DO THIS POSE	Those with high blood pressure, detached retina, glaucoma, or hiatal hernia. Those with injuries to the neck that would be exacerbated by increased weight through the cervical vertebrae. Do not practice if you are menstruating.
PRENATAL SUGGESTIONS	
HAVING TROUBLE?	The area around my kidneys aches while in the pose.
TRY . . .	*This may be because of weakness or chronic tension in the mid-back. Try practicing Bridge Pose (page 194) and Shoulder Stand before coming into Plow. Raise your feet onto a chair, and lower them onto the floor only when you can do so without discomfort.*

Knee-to-Ear Pose (*Karnapidasana*)

You'll Need

> A few blankets
> A bolster

Here's How

Beginners: For retreating from the hubbub of the world, it's hard to beat the enfolded fetal position of Knee-to-Ear Pose. Curling the body inward shifts us from the "acting-and-doing" state into the "feeling-and-being" state. The practice of containing one's energy develops a sense of security and safety. Giving yourself this psychological boundary helps build reserves, so that you can more effectively extend outward into life with boundlessness.

If you are new to this pose, you can practice a variation of the full posture by taking Plow Pose first with your feet supported on a chair (page 226). Have a bolster by your side and, when you are ready to transition into Knee-to-Ear Pose, push the chair away and replace it with a bolster. Slowly bend your knees and lower them to rest on the bolster. Raising your legs will reduce the flexion on your spine and neck and make relaxing easier for you. To release your shoulders, interlock your hands behind your back and extend them strongly away from your neck and down into the floor (Figure 222). Then place your hands on your back, encouraging the breath to move into your back against the pressure of your palms. Stay for one minute or more, enjoying the experience of being enfolded. When you are ready to come down, support your back with your hands and slowly roll out.

Advanced: For advanced practice in which your knees come to rest on the floor on either side of the ears, I recommend using only two blankets and moving back so that your head and neck are resting on the blanket as well. If you use more blankets, you are creating an extra artificial distance between your knees and the floor. Bringing your head and neck onto the blanket may seem contradictory to previous directions, but this pose is structurally quite different from Shoulder Stand or Plow in that the back is flexed rather than extended. It usually feels more natural to allow the neck to follow this natural flexion, but if this is not comfortable, feel free to work with the head and neck off the blankets.

It usually feels best to enter full Knee-to-Ear Pose toward the end of an inversion practice, as it has a deeply calming and releasing effect. You can come into it either directly from Shoulder Stand or from Plow. In the final stages the knees will rest on the floor, pressing lightly against the ears. The tops of the feet will rest on the floor behind the head. Close your eyes and allow your attention to move inward. Focus on breathing into the back of your body while allowing the abdomen to fold back toward the spine. Fold the arms over the backs of the knees

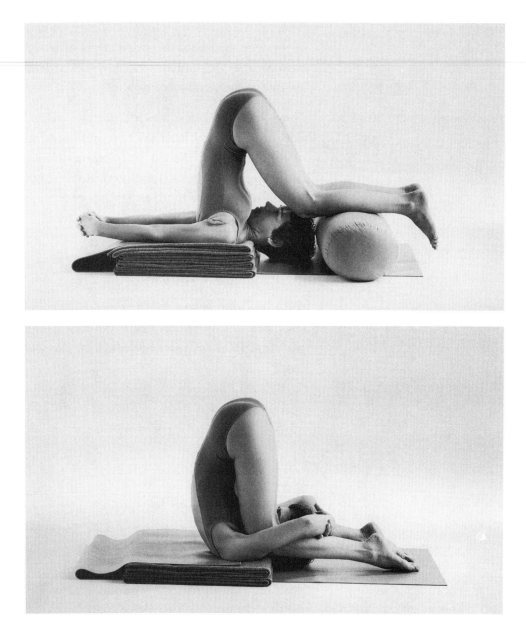

FIGURE 222

FIGURE 223

to complete the pose and stay for one to three minutes, continuing to breathe softly into the back (Figure 223). Another wonderful variation is to rest the knee and upper shin on your face against the orbits of the eyes. Applying this gentle pressure to these sensitive points releases deeply held tension within and around your eyes and face, and can be an easier position to hold than the full flexion of the final pose.

When you are ready to come down, roll out very slowly, resting with your knees bent. After this deep flexion it usually feels good to take Revolved Belly Pose (page 162) briefly on each side. Take the time to enjoy the afterglow of this remarkable posture by resting for a bit in deep relaxation before you go on with your day.

BENEFITS AND EFFECTS	Releases the spinal muscles and relaxes tension in the legs. Increases the circulation of blood through the abdominal area. Induces a deep sense of security and relaxation.
WHO SHOULDN'T DO THIS POSE	Those with high blood pressure, detached retina, glaucoma, or hiatal hernia. Those with injuries to the neck that would be exacerbated by increased weight through the cervical vertebrae, and those with disc injuries. Do not practice if you are menstruating.
PRENATAL SUGGESTIONS	
HAVING TROUBLE?	My breathing feels restricted.
TRY . . .	*Soften the area around the front of the groin and thigh, and allow your abdomen to fall back toward your spine. Focus on expanding your breath into your back.*

VII
Restorative Postures and Breathing Practices

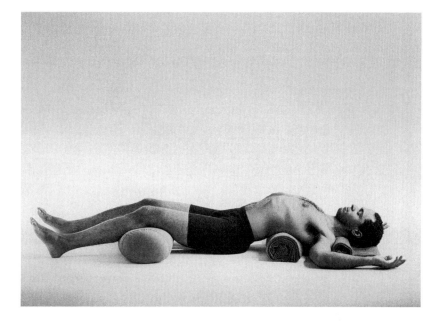

INTRODUCTION

*O*ne of the oldest and most beloved prayers from the Vedic tradition, the *Gayatri Mantra,* tells us that all of life is sustained by one ever-renewing source. When we practice restorative postures, what we are restoring is our connection with the part of our mind that is linked with this enduring, vast, and silent source. Yoga tells us that when we are in intimate connection with this part of our mind and thus tapped into a greater mind, we are also tuned in to the body's natural ability to heal itself.

While restorative postures are ideal for those times when we feel depleted or when we are recovering from an illness, I encourage the reader to consider a proactive approach and to make restoratives a regular part of your yoga practice. Reserving one practice a week for these rejuvenators or including a few in each day's practice will help build stores of energy that can prevent conditions of depletion and can pave the way toward sustainable health. The breathing practices presented in this chapter offer additional support for rejuvenation and can be done in conjunction with the restoratives, as a part of a normal yoga practice, or on their own.

What makes a restorative posture different from other yoga poses? First, most restorative postures are adaptations of classic yoga postures, during the practice of which you are *passively supported* by props such as chairs, blankets, or bolsters. Because you are supported you do not have to *use* energy to *get* energy. You place yourself in a position to *receive* energy. Second, the poses are practiced with the body in a deliberately *mild* or graduated version of the classic pose, focusing less on stretching muscles and more on releasing tension and increasing the circulation of blood to key organs and glands. In a restorative posture that has been well propped, one feels absolutely comfortable with no intense stretching sensations. Don't mistake this, however, with a mild result. It is the graduated nature of the position that will allow you to stay for much *longer periods* of time than you might normally if you were practicing a posture more actively. This longer stay allows key organs and glands to become drenched with revitalizing blood. Because the action reaches deep into the nervous system, the practice of these postures can dismantle chronic tension patterns, improve immune function, and bring the body and mind back to their original state of equilibrium.

To the untrained eye, these postures seem easy. Don't be mistaken—these are some of the most sophisticated postures in the yoga repertoire. A newcomer to yoga who is accustomed to seeking strong sensation in the muscles as proof that "something is happening" will need to look deeper to feel for the more subtle physiological and psychological effects. It was only when my own health was compromised by a bad case of mononucleosis many years ago that I discovered how amazing these postures can be for restoring health. The angle and precise position of each part of the body is crucial for these postures to work their magic, so I recommend that you seek the help of a practitioner experienced in their use to check your practice.

The development of many of these postures is credited to B. K. S. Iyengar, of Pune, India. Judith Lasater's comprehensive book *Relax and Renew* is an excellent resource for exploring restoratives in more depth.

KEY MOVING PRINCIPLES FOR RESTORATIVE POSTURES AND BREATHING PRACTICES

1. BREATHE
Let the Breath Move You

2. YIELD
Yield to the Earth: Weight and Levity

3. ENGAGE
Engage the Whole Body: Focus on Cellular Respiration

ESSENTIAL SKILLS

Lying Down and Getting Up with Ease

Although coming onto and off of the floor sounds like the simplest of tasks, it is a task we do many times in our yoga practice, and thus it forms a bridge between one movement and another. These transitional movements allow us to carry the relaxation and focus of one moment into the next, an especially important skill to learn when practicing restoratives. Most people perform this everyday transitional movement in a way that is jarring on the lower back and neck and stressful to the back muscles. Take the time in the following inquiry to discover the pleasure of moving onto and off the earth with ease.

～ INQUIRY ～

Lying Down and Getting Up with Ease

Most people get up off the floor by lifting from the head, neck, and spinal muscles. In this inquiry you'll learn how to use your limbs for support so these vulnerable areas can stay soft and released. This is an especially important skill if you have any preexisting back problems, because the transition into and out of postures (whether getting out of bed or the car) can strain and even provoke a muscle spasm if done without the support of your arms and legs.

First let's learn how to come onto the floor. Sit with your feet folded to your right side with your weight resting primarily on your left buttock. Slowly slide your left hand out along the floor away from your head, turning your head and chest to look toward the floor. Use your right arm to steady your descent, making

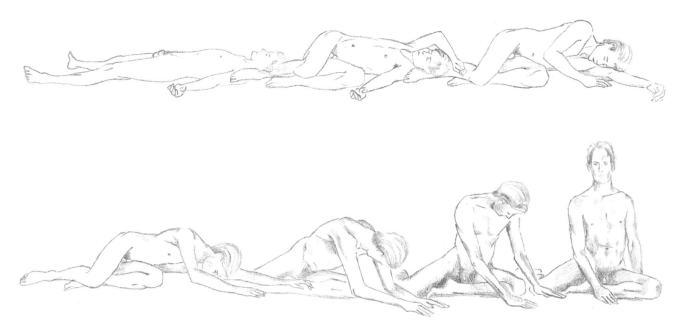

FIGURE 225

sure you find your support from your arms while keeping the head, neck, and spinal column relaxed. Slide the left arm out until you are resting on your left armpit, and then slowly roll onto the outside of your left shoulder and follow the circular action of the motion to roll all the way onto your back.

Now slowly extend your legs out along the floor into Corpse Pose. To transition back to sitting, you reverse the sequence of movements. First, bend your left knee and then the right and roll onto your left side. Continue to roll your body until your forehead is facing the floor and your right hand has come to rest on the floor beside your head. Let your head and neck drape passively as you press your right hand into the floor, simultaneously bringing your left hand underneath your chest. Here's the trick: Use the push of your arms to draw yourself up without tensing through your neck and back muscles. Slowly curl up to sitting, letting your neck and head be the last part of the spine to come upright (Figure 225).

Practice rolling onto and off of the floor until the action feels smooth, seamless, and circular and you can remain relaxed throughout the movement.

Corpse Pose (*Savasana*)

Corpse Pose is said to be one of the most difficult postures to master. Far from taking a chance to kick back, we learn how to enter a state of profound relaxation while remaining conscious and attentive—a state of mind quite unfamiliar to the average person. To enter this state we practice a kind of conscious dying, a letting go of the things that make us feel armored and separate and, thus, that cause us to suffer and to accumulate tension. First we let go of the effort of our practice, already past. Then we let go of physical tension which, in the yogic way of thinking, is nothing more than the accumulation of ideas and attitudes that are being repeated unconsciously day after day. These habitual thought patterns cause tension to accumulate and to be held in the tissues of the body. As we consciously relinquish the attachments we have to our image, our responsibilities, our problems, our opinions, and our likes and dislikes, we go through a process very similar to the one that we will all face when we die. This letting go allows us to pare away the trappings of who we think we are to get to the core of that part of our self that continues beyond the death of the body. Suspended in this blissful state where all our worries and tensions have melted away, we allow ourselves to rest completely. At the end of the practice we roll over on our sides into a fetal position, symbolizing the possibility that we can begin each day anew without the weight of these attachments dragging us down. Ultimately the practice is about learning to be in Corpse Pose all the time so we don't go through our days letting unimportant things stick to us like tar and feathers.

My beginning students find this one of the most pleasurable postures and seem to learn the Sanskrit for this posture quicker than any other! Corpse Pose is one of the four motif movements in the family of yoga *asanas,* and its practice underlies all the other restorative postures.

∽ INQUIRY ∽

Corpse Pose

You'll Need

> 2 to 3 blankets
> An eye bag

Here's How

Roll out a blanket the length of your body. Sit with your knees bent in front of you with your feet hips-width apart. Look down between your feet and check that your feet are equidistant from each other and your legs are not veering to one side. It's important to lie as symmetrically as possible, as this will enhance your relaxation and ensure that energy is allowed to circulate equally throughout the body. Now lean back on your elbows and slowly straighten your legs along the floor, checking again that the legs have not strayed to the left or right. Place your thumbs against the tops of your buttocks and slowly drag your buttocks over your thumbs, drawing the skin of your buttocks down toward your heels to lengthen your lower back. As you recline, place your lower, then middle, then upper rib cage on the floor. Place a folded blanket underneath your head and neck, raising your head so that your forehead is slightly higher than your chin. This will draw the gaze of the eyes downward into the heart, helping you to move your attention inward. Spread the arms away from the body so there is air between your armpits and your upper arms, and turn your palms upward. Make sure that you are warm, and if necessary cover yourself with a blanket (it's best to do this as you are reclining to avoid having to readjust your position). If you wish, cover your eyes with an eye bag (Figure 226).

There are many ways that you can guide yourself in *Savasana*. It's helpful to attend yoga classes to be able to receive this guidance first from a teacher. The following is one of my favorite visualizations. It centers on relaxing tension in the face and head and using this local release to affect a global sense of relaxation in the rest of the body. I hope you enjoy it.

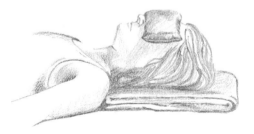

FIGURE 226

Let your attention come to rest lightly on your face. Allow your features and any expression that you hold to soften. Beginning with the eyes, release the skin around the orbits of the eyes and allow the eyes to become like still pools of water. Let your gaze turn inward and down, as if looking at the bottom of this still pool. Consciously release the skin on your forehead downward and out toward the temples. As you come to the temples, allow the jaw to open slightly, feeling the joint hanging loose and slack. As you release the jaw, go inside the mouth and open the space from the inside of the jaw on one side to the inside of the jaw on the other side. With this new spaciousness in the mouth, swallow a few times and relax the throat, allowing the back of the throat to become hollow. Feeling inside the mouth, let the cheeks grow slack, the tongue pressing neither on the teeth nor on the roof of the mouth. Soften the skin of your lips, and as your lips part slightly, consciously let the skin over your entire face grow loose, as if it were draped like a soft blanket over your face. Now let the scalp release its grip on your skull, and as the scalp grows slack feel the back of the skull broadening on the floor. Let this broadness extend down your neck. As you let go of the effort of maintaining your image, allow this relaxation in your face to move inward. Let it move easily and completely down into your brain until the brain itself feels completely relaxed. As the brain relaxes, let this relaxation you feel in your brain travel throughout your entire body. Let it travel deeply into the core of your body and into all your limbs, through your arms to your fingers and through your legs to your toes.

Now let go of any effort and enjoy this deep relaxation for at least ten minutes. When you feel refreshed, slowly roll over on your side and come up to sitting. Take a few minutes to reacclimate yourself, being careful not to jump back into the world of work and worry too quickly. Know that you can carry this relaxation with you throughout the day wherever you go.

QUIET EYES . . . QUIET MIND

During the practice of restorative postures, the eyes remain closed. Closing the eyes draws the attention inward, eliminates normal visual stimulation, and blocks out light. Closing the eyelids, however, does not necessarily mean the eyes themselves have become relaxed or still. It is not until the gaze turns inward to see "inside" that the outward-moving projections of the mind can begin to curve back in a self-reflective way. There are two yoga accessories that can deeply facilitate this stilling of the eyes and the relaxation of the mind that accompanies it.

The first is an eye bag (page 28). Whenever you are in a reclining position, you can use the eye bag to shield the eyes from light, and the slight weight of the bag to release tension around the eyes themselves. The other accessory, although less familiar to many, is an elastic bandage (page 28). The elastic bandage not only blocks out light but provides a firm pressure around the frontalis and temporalis muscles of the forehead and temples, as well as the scalp at the back of the head (Figure 227). Relaxation in these muscles has been shown to relieve the symptoms of headaches.[1]

Once you are familiar with and confident in practicing the restorative postures, you can use an eye bandage during your practice to accelerate and deepen the effects of the practice. During times of intense work pressure or when there are just too many things happening in my own life, I do my entire practice with the eyes covered, from standing postures to

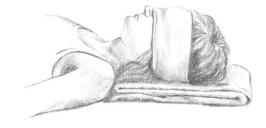

FIGURE 227

Corpse Pose. Working for longer periods of time with the eyes covered brings about a profound sensitivity to inner sensations often missed when the attention is focused on the surrounding environment or even the external form of one's own body. At the end of my practice I am amazed at how the creases around my forehead, eyes, and the corners of my mouth have softened or even disappeared, and how my face has resumed a youthful appearance.

∾ INQUIRY ∾

Practicing with the Eye Bag and Eye Bandage

You'll Need

> One eye bag
> An elastic bandage
> (*Remove eyeglasses or contact lenses before doing this practice.*)

Unroll an elastic bandage about 6 inches. Hold the end with one hand and start by covering the back of your head. Wind the bandage around your head, making sure it is not so tight that it is pulling on the skin of your forehead and temples or placing undue pressure on the eyes themselves. When you have wrapped the length of the bandage, fold it under on the side of your head rather than the back, where it may produce a bump that will prevent your head from resting evenly on the floor. If you need to see to enter, leave, or adjust your posture, simply fold the bottom portion of the bandage up over the eyes for a moment. As much as possible, however, attempt to have everything you need at hand so you can work uninterrupted with the eyes covered. Lie back into Corpse Pose and spend at least ten minutes sensing and feeling the difference the eye bandage makes to your relaxation.

Some people thoroughly enjoy the use of the eye bandage, while others find it makes them feel claustrophobic—use it only if it's comfortable for you. When you are finished, slowly unwind the eye bandage (rather than pulling it off the head) as this will gradually release the pressure on the forehead, bringing you slowly back to the outer world.

THE RESTORATIVE POSTURES

Variations on Corpse Pose

Many people do not find lying flat on the back entirely comfortable. Experiment with these variations until you find a position that allows you to relax for at least five minutes without having to move.

You'll Need

A chair
A bolster or 3 to 4 blankets
A sandbag (or a bag of rice or beans)

Here's How

Variation with a Chair

Place your lower legs on the seat of a folding chair. Your lower leg should lie parallel to the floor—if it doesn't and your heels are lifted off of the chair, raise your back on the floor with a few folded blankets. This is an adjustment that smaller people will need to make. Place a folded blanket under your head and neck, and cover your eyes. Place a sandbag or bag of rice on your lower abdomen. This will help soften and release tension in your abdomen and encourage you to breathe more deeply into the belly (Figure 228).

Variation with Bolster

Fold a blanket into a cylinder or use a round bolster. Place the bolster underneath your knees and raise your heels with another folded blanket. This last adjustment will make a huge difference to the feeling of release in your lower back. Place a folded blanket under your head and neck, and cover your eyes (Figure 229).

Downward-Facing Corpse Pose

When we lie on our back, the surface of the body that is in contact with the earth increases in tone. This stimulates the sympathetic nervous system—the part of your nervous system responsible for fight-or-flight responses. I am sure the yogis were aware of this, as lying on the back encourages a certain level of attentiveness. When we lie on the front of the body, this increases the tone through the soft organs and stimulates the parasympathetic nervous system—the part of the nervous system responsible for functions such as breathing and digestion. Many people find this variation deeply soothing, and it is especially helpful for people who breathe high up in the chest, with the excess tension in the neck, shoulders, and upper back that accompanies chronic chest breathing.

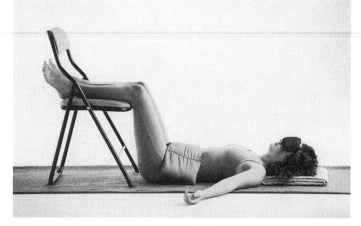

FIGURE 228

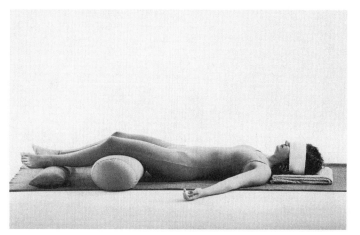

FIGURE 229

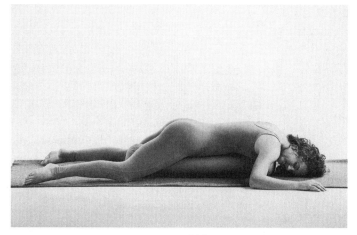

FIGURE 230

Place a large bolster or a stack of folded blankets on top of a well-padded surface. Lie with your belly and chest supported on the bolster, with your head, legs, and arms draped over the sides onto the floor. Let your head and neck cascade over the end of the bolster, and rest your forehead on the floor. Alternatively, turn your head gently to the side if this is comfortable for you (Figure 230). If you have no preexisting neck problems, you can do Downward-Facing Corpse Pose with your entire body resting on the floor, but this requires a more intense rotation through the neck. Try the posture with and without the bolster to see which is most effective. Enjoy!

BENEFITS AND EFFECTS	Releases physical and mental tension. Improves immune function. Allows the body to heal itself.
WHO SHOULDN'T DO THIS POSE	☺
PRENATAL SUGGESTIONS	After the first trimester it is no longer safe to lie flat on the back. You can do a most effective Corpse Pose lying on your side with a pillow under your head, in between your knees, and behind your back.
HAVING TROUBLE?	My hips and lower back hurt in all the variations. I even have trouble sleeping at night.
TRY . . .	*This level of pain is a sign that you need to seek professional help. When there is constant pain that remains unchanged no matter what position you are in, it can be a sign of an organic problem such as a kidney infection or abdominal abscess.*

Supported Forward Bend

You can practice almost any forward bend with your forehead supported on a chair or bolster. Supported forward bends move the energy down out of the head and deep into the pelvis, increasing the circulation of blood throughout the organs of digestion and reproduction. Your neck, shoulders, and back relax as your attention shifts into your lower body, and symptoms of headache and eyestrain are alleviated.

You'll Need

A few blankets
A chair or bolster

Here's How

Sit with your legs crossed, raising your pelvis on a folded blanket if necessary. Place a chair in front of you (secure it on a mat or position the chair against a wall), and slowly tip forward, resting your forehead on the edge of the chair. Pad the edge of the chair with a folded towel if it is hard, and cross your forearms above your head. Make sure that the front of your body is relaxed and long. If bringing your head down to the level of the chair causes strong stretching sensations in your back or hips, raise the height of the seat with cushions until you can stay comfortably. Alternatively, if you are a more advanced student, you can experiment with supporting your head lower down with a bolster. Additionally, if you suffer from shoulder tension, try placing a sandbag across the top of your shoulders (Figure 231)—most people find this feels amazing!

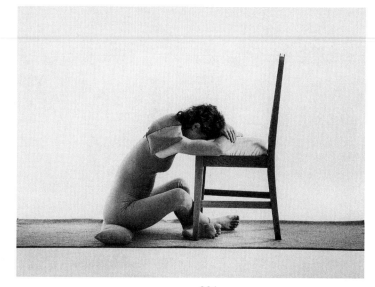

FIGURE 231

Breathe low and slow into your belly, drawing your attention inward and down. Imagine that your breath is like a plow moving through hard soil, turning and loosening the soil of your body as you work progressively downward from the back of your neck, through the muscles either side of your spine, to your tailbone. Stay for three to five minutes and then change the cross of your legs and arms and practice on the second side.

You Can Practice These Forward Bends in a Similar Way

Head-to-Knee Pose (page 143)

Wide-Spread-Angle Pose I and II (page 146)

BENEFITS AND EFFECTS	Releases eye, neck, and shoulder tension. Improves digestive function. Tones and helps regulate sexual function.
WHO SHOULDN'T DO THIS POSE	Those with disc problems should be cautious.
PRENATAL SUGGESTIONS	⊛
HAVING TROUBLE?	My knees hurt in all the positions.
TRY . . .	*Raise your pelvis higher on folded blankets, and then place a folded blanket underneath each knee.*

Breathing-Easy Position

This position is ideal for opening and releasing tension in your diaphragm, chest, and shoulders. Because it raises the chest and diaphragm slightly above the height of the abdominal organs, it makes breathing easier. This position can be used during almost all the breathing practices at the end of this chapter and is especially

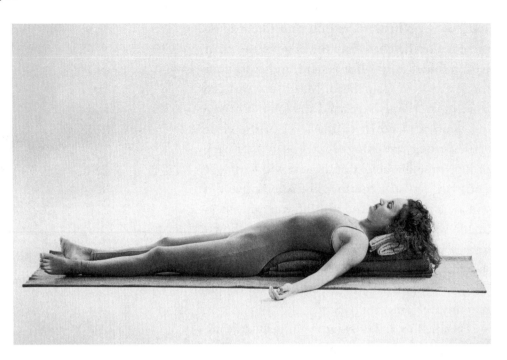

FIGURE 232

soothing when the sinuses and lungs are congested. Experiment with the height of the prop until you find a position that feels comfortable for your back.

You'll Need

3 to 5 blankets

Here's How

Fold two blankets into a bolster shape, about 3 inches high, 8 to 10 inches wide, and at least 3 feet long. Lie with your buttocks on the floor and slowly recline, being careful that your spine is symmetrical along the length of the bolster. Bend your knees and lift your pelvis briefly, drawing the buttocks under so that the lower back is long and released. Then extend the legs straight, letting them rest about a foot apart. Raise the head with a folded blanket until the forehead is slightly higher than the chin (Figure 232). You can rest in this position for five to ten minutes (or longer if you are completely comfortable).

If you have blocked sinuses or congestion in your lungs, try raising the bolster height to 5 inches or more. When you do this, your arms will tend to hang at a sharp angle from the chest. Support each arm with a pillow so that there is a smooth transition from your chest through to each hand.

BENEFITS AND EFFECTS   Releases tension in the diaphragm, chest, and shoulders. Facilitates diaphragmatic breathing. Helps clear congestion from sinuses and lungs.

WHO SHOULDN'T DO THIS POSE   ☺

PRENATAL SUGGESTIONS	(symbol) After the first trimester you must raise the chest so that you are at a 30-degree angle or more (see page 85).
HAVING TROUBLE?	My lower back feels uncomfortable.
TRY . . .	*Try lowering the height of the blankets to just 2 or 3 inches. Additionally, you can add a small roll underneath your knees.*

Supported Bound-Angle Pose
(*Salamba Supta Baddha Konasana*)

This posture is considered by many to be one of the most powerful positions for regulating and balancing a woman's menstrual cycle and the symptoms associated with premenstrual tension, menstrual cramps, and menopausal syndromes. Blood flow is directed into the pelvis, bathing the reproductive organs and glands and helping to balance hormone function. We have had positive results in alleviating the pain of prostatitis with male students at our studio, which makes us believe that it may have a rejuvenative effect on the male reproductive system as well.

There are myriad ways to practice Supported Bound-Angle Pose. Your back can be raised slightly or at a steeper angle during pregnancy (see page 85 for prenatal cautions). In other variations your back remains on the floor with the feet and lower legs raised. In still other versions your back is gently arched over a small cylindrical bolster placed at a right angle to the spine. Below I have shown the classic variation of this posture.

You'll Need

> 3 to 5 blankets
> An eye bag if you have one

Here's How

Fold two or three blankets so that they form a rectangular bolster about 8 inches wide, 4 inches high, and at least 3 feet long. Sit with your buttocks on the floor directly in front of the bolster and bring the soles of your feet together so that your legs form a diamond shape. Reclining onto your elbows, lie back onto the bolster, being careful to center your spine. Place a folded blanket underneath each thigh so that your legs are fully supported and you do not feel any pulling in your inner groin, thighs, or hips. Also place a pillow or folded blanket under each arm so there is a smooth transition rather than a sharp drop-off from your chest through to your hands. Raise your head slightly on a folded towel so that your forehead is a little higher than your chin, and then release your shoulders back so that your arms extend with the palms up (Figure 233). Cover your eyes with an eye bag.

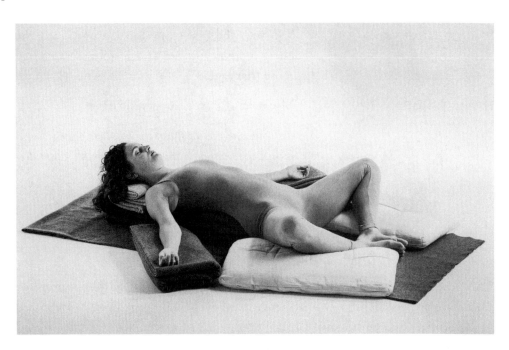

FIGURE 233

From this position let the pull of gravity release your hips and inner thighs. Focus your attention on your abdomen and in through the pelvic floor, softening and relaxing with each breath cycle. If the room is cool, cover yourself with a blanket and stay for five to ten minutes. When you are ready to come out, use your hands to raise one knee and roll over onto your side. Take a few moments to collect yourself before sitting up.

BENEFITS AND EFFECTS	Releases tension in the inner groin, pelvic floor, and hips. Opens the abdominal organs. Nourishes the digestive and reproductive systems.
WHO SHOULDN'T DO THIS POSE	People with sacroiliac problems should be careful to prop the legs so that they are the same height on both sides.
PRENATAL SUGGESTIONS	After the first trimester you must raise the angle of the bolster so that your abdomen is at a 30-degree angle or more. Some women find crossing the legs rather than bringing the soles of the feet together more comfortable for the lower back.
HAVING TROUBLE?	My lower back aches.
TRY . . .	*If lowering the height of the blanket does not eliminate your discomfort, try practicing the posture with your back on the floor and your feet and lower legs raised about 6 inches onto a bolster.*

The Great Rejuvenator (*Viparita Karani*)

This is one of the most powerful and most useful of all the restorative postures. If you have time for no other practice, I recommend this one. The Great Rejuvenator is remarkably similar to Shoulder Stand and has an amazing ability to neutralize the body—if you are feeling tired, it tends to boost your energy, and if you come to your practice with the jumps and jitters, it brings you down to earth.

You'll Need

A cylindrical bolster or 3 to 4 blankets
A yoga tie
An eye bag
A wall

Here's How

Fold the blankets so they form a rectangular bolster about 6 to 10 inches high, about 10 inches wide, and at least 3 feet long (or use a cylindrical bolster). People who are very flexible or who have long torsos should have a higher and wider prop. Place the bolster lengthwise along a wall, leaving about a 2-inch gap between the bolster and the wall.

Sit on one end of the bolster and carefully roll onto your side so that your right hip is supported on the bolster and your right shoulder is on the floor (Figure 234). Using your right arm for support, roll your body so that your buttocks are on the bolster with your legs extended straight up the wall, and with your shoulders, head, and neck resting on the floor. Your chin will be drawn slightly down toward your chest. In the final position your hips will be very close to, if not touching, the wall; your abdomen will be parallel to the floor; and your chest and spine will cascade in a rounded arch over the bolster (Figure 235). Imagine the pose like a series of waterfalls: your legs are the first waterfall, with the fluid pooling in the basin of the belly; your chest and spine are the second waterfall, with fluid pooling in the throat and upper chest. Many people find that tying the ankles or upper third of the thighs together allows them to relax their legs more completely.

If your hamstrings and back are very stiff, you may have the feeling that you are sliding off the bolster. Instead of a cascade there will be a straight line from the hips to the shoulders. When this happens, all the fluid from the legs and pelvis pours down the body directly into your head, causing a feeling of pressure around your forehead, temples, and eyes. Additionally, because the abdominal organs are at an angle, they will slide up into the diaphragm, making it *harder* rather than easier to breathe freely (Figure 236). If necessary, move the bolster farther away from the wall and allow your legs to be at a slight angle to the wall (which is easier on those tight hamstrings). You might also experiment with lowering or raising the height of your bolster, or folding a blanket into a wedge shape and placing it on the bolster so that the narrow edge faces the wall. This will help to tip your pelvis and hips

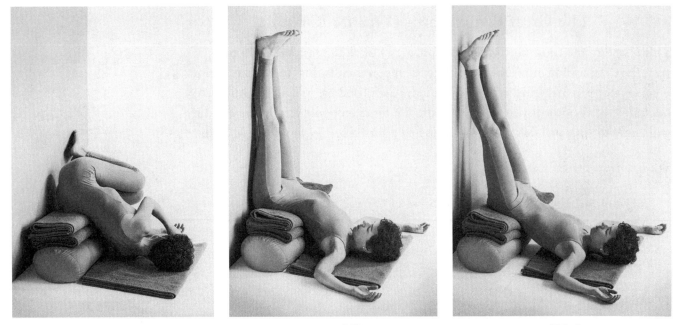

FIGURE 234   FIGURE 235   FIGURE 236. *Incorrect*

back toward the wall. Be willing to come down and adjust your propping. The small initial investment of time required to find the best propping is insignificant compared to the powerful restorative effect of this pose when it is practiced correctly. Once you have found an arrangement that is comfortable, make note of it for future reference.

Relax completely for five to fifteen minutes. Observe the subtle shift of your internal physiology: the deepening of your breath, the slowing of the heartbeat, the quieting of the mind. When you are ready to come out, slowly bend your knees and push yourself away from the wall until your back is flat on the floor. Cross your ankles and rest them on the bolster for a few minutes before rolling onto your side and sitting up.

BENEFITS AND EFFECTS	Reduces water retention in the ankles and legs, and flushes the legs of lactic acid buildup. Excellent for post-athletic activity or after long periods standing. Balances the neuroendocrine system. Facilitates deep breathing.
WHO SHOULDN'T DO THIS POSE	Those with hiatal hernias, eye pressure, retinal problems, and heart or neck problems. Menstruating women and those with spondylolisthesis and spondylolysis. Additionally, those with high blood pressure should be cautious. Those with high blood pressure controlled by medication may try a reduced variation with the pelvis level

on the ground and gradually raise the height of the pelvis over a period of time if this causes no problems. Paradoxically, practice of this pose can help regulate blood pressure over time but should be attempted only under supervision.

PRENATAL SUGGESTIONS

HAVING TROUBLE?   I feel discomfort in my lower back.

TRY . . .   *Practice with the pelvis flat on the floor and the legs up the wall. Gradually raise the pelvis over a period of time.*

BREATHING PRACTICES

The following practices can be done at the end of a restorative session or at the end of any practice session after the body is relaxed and the mind quiet. These practices help to refine the quality of the breath and serve to repattern the nervous system at a very deep level. For a more detailed discussion of breathing and breathing practices, refer to *The Breathing Book*, by Donna Farhi.

Straw Breathing[2]

You'll Need

A straw
2 blankets, if you are reclining in the Breathing-Easy position
A chair or cushion, if you are sitting

Purpose

This is one of the most powerful techniques I know for reteaching the body to breathe primarily from the diaphragm. Because diaphragmatic breathing is controlled at a level below the conscious mind, when we "try" to change the breath the mind does not have the necessary skills to go about this deep neuromuscular repatterning and thus usually resorts to willful and mechanical efforts. Rather than attempting to change the breath from this vantage point, in straw breathing we simply place a small obstacle in the breath's way, an obstacle that requires the body to figure out a new and more effective way of breathing. In this way we bypass the mind and let the body reorient itself in its own time. Usually people halve their breaths per minute within three to five minutes of straw breathing—obtaining this remarkable result without any feeling of strain. It is a particularly good technique for chronic chest breathers and for those with asthma who tend to curtail their exhalations.

Here's How

Recline in the Breathing-Easy position (page 241) or sit on a cushion or chair. Before you begin straw breathing do a check-in with your breath and count how many breath cycles you take per minute. Once you've established this baseline, place a long straw in your mouth and hold on to it gently with your hands. Don't try to hold it without the help of your hands, or you will unnecessarily contract your facial and jaw muscles. Breathe *in* through your nose and then breathe *out* through your mouth into the straw, working gently so as not to push the breath out. When you take your next breath in, lightly touch your tongue to the roof of your mouth to prevent yourself from breathing in through your mouth. Continue for three minutes. At the end of each exhalation allow the inhalation to arise spontaneously. When the diaphragm initiates the inhalation it will feel like a gentle "bounce" up through the center of your body. If you can allow this to happen, the incoming breath will be effortless. We usually don't trust this to happen and jump in prematurely by initiating the inhalation with our upper chest and shoulders. Toward the end of your three-minute session, again count the number of breath cycles per minutes. Has it changed? Over time you can increase your straw-breathing sessions to seven to ten minutes.

A word of warning: Some people feel a sense of panic when they first try the straw inquiry. I believe this is because increasing the length of the exhalation is "counterintuitive"; that is, we're convinced we have to put the emphasis on the inhalation or we won't get enough air. If you feel uncomfortable, just stop and take a few normal breaths until you again feel relaxed and calm. I encourage you to persevere, because the results of this wonderful technique are truly dramatic.

The Purifying Breath (*Nadi Shodhanam*)

You'll Need

A cushion or chair to sit on

Purpose

Nadi Shodhanam, or "alternate nostril breathing," is a sophisticated practice in which you deliberately change the flow of air through the nostrils to balance your psychophysiology. The yogis believe that when the right nostril is open the *surya,* or sun/heating element, is dominant, and that when the left nostril is open the *chandra,* or moon/cooling element, is dominant. By opening and closing the nostrils in varying patterns one can adjust the physiology of the body much like regulating a hot and cold faucet to produce warm water. Although present research on the subject is controversial, many believe that right-nostril dominance stimulates the arousal-producing sympathetic nervous system and left-nostril dominance elicits the relaxation-producing parasympathetic system.[3] By alternating the flow of air in a regulated way, yogis create an equilibrium in the two branches of the autonomic nervous systems and a balance between excitation and relaxation. This is an excellent practice for centering the mind, especially before a potentially stressful or challenging event.

Here's How

Sit cross-legged on a cushion or sit on a chair if you find this more comfortable. Using the left or the right hand (it's good to alternate hands each time you practice), fold the index and third finger inward to touch the palm near the base of the thumb. Bring the thumb and tip of the ring finger together to touch. Let the little finger rest gently against the side of the ring finger.

Bow your head slightly downward, as if you were going to put a hood over your head. As you make the gesture downward, let your awareness curve back into itself, cultivating a self-reflective state. Bring your hand up, open the thumb and ring finger, and place the tip of the thumb on the side of one nostril and the tip of the ring finger on the other nostril. The cycle is as follows:

1. Close the left nostril and exhale completely through the right nostril.
2. Inhale through the right nostril.
3. Close the right nostril and exhale through the left nostril.
4. Inhale through the left nostril.
5. Close the left nostril and exhale through the right nostril. This completes one cycle. Continue for up to twenty cycles, finishing by exhaling through the right nostril.

As you proceed with the cycles be careful that your hand is not pulling the head off center. Also check that you are not slouching forward with your chest. Let your fingers be sensitive so that as you close a nostril you are not pressing so hard that the septum is being pushed off center.

Once you have become adept at the basic form of alternate nostril breathing, you can begin to time each segment of the breath by mentally counting. In this way, the inhalation and exhalation will be exactly the same length. Start with a number that is absolutely comfortable, such as four, and gradually build up to six, eight, ten, and even twelve counts for each phase of the breath. Do not increase the length of the count if you have even the slightest sensation of strain or discomfort.

The Pacifying Breath (*Viloma* II)

You'll Need

2 to 3 blankets for the Breathing-Easy position

Purpose

In this practice you trick the body into lengthening the exhalation by dividing the exhalation into three parts, pausing briefly after each successive exhalation. The combination of the staggered exhalation and the pauses in between create a longer exhalation than you might normally make. This lengthened exhalation in turn stimulates a deepening of the inhalation. This is an especially helpful practice to do if you have difficulty falling asleep. It is also an effective technique for diminishing anxiety that doesn't seem to have any particular source, and for those times when there is a buildup of tension in the body, as often happens before the menses or during menopause.

Here's How

Assume the Breathing-Easy position or simply lie on your back with your knees bent. Spend a few minutes to settle yourself consciously relax the body. To begin the exercise, take a normal breath in and then divide the exhalation into three equal parts, pausing very briefly between them. It will sound something like this:

Inhalation
exhale-pause,
exhale-pause,
exhale-pause,
Inhalation
One or two normal breaths in and out, then repeat from beginning.

If you have a very weak respiratory capacity, you may need to take more normal breaths in and out between cycles. Then begin again, inhaling, followed by a staggered exhalation, letting each part of the exhalation be the same length as the others. The pause should be a moment of suspension as when you say "ah," rather than a feeling of contracting or holding the breath. If you feel short of breath, you are probably trying to make the exhalation or pauses too long. Adjust until you feel completely relaxed, with no sense of grabbing for the inhalation. Also make sure that you are not breathing in or out during the pause.

You may find that images can help you create a smooth, even rhythm. I like to picture the breath movement as a waterfall flowing down, collecting in a pool during the pause, and then flowing down to the next pool. Or you can imagine that you are descending a tall ladder, exhaling as you step down, pausing at each step, and then descending farther. Continue with this practice for a total of about ten cycles and then completely relax. Take a few minutes to feel the effects of your practice before you continue with your day.

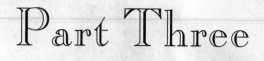

Part Three
~
Practice

VIII
Putting It All Together

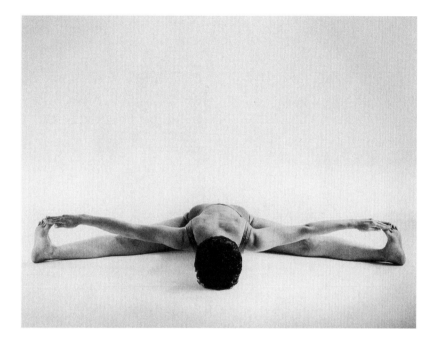

INTRODUCTION

*C*reating a balanced yoga practice is like learning to cook a good meal. Before you can cook intuitively you first need to build some basic skills, and for this you require clear instructions, a list of ingredients, set measurements, and, if possible, the help of someone who is a competent cook. Once the basics are mastered, you then have the freedom to experiment with spices and unusual flavor combinations without too much risk of an indigestible result. Similarly, when you begin to put a home practice together, it is helpful to follow a set, structured sequence. This will help you develop a solid foundation of skills and give you the confidence so necessary for establishing a routine. After basic sequences have been mastered and the habit of practice is well developed, you can begin to work more intuitively, trusting that the reservoir of information you have stored through your practice will guide you toward a balanced result.

To take the analogy further, consider each *asana* as you would the individual ingredients in a recipe. How an ingredient tastes and the effect it has in the body is always in relationship to the whole recipe. Garlic has a different effect depending on whether you use it raw or cooked, and what you combine with that garlic will further modify its properties. In the same way, the yoga *asanas* are a relational system. The postures that precede and follow each *asana* have an enormous influence on the overall effect that posture has within your practice. As you become familiar with the inner workings of each *asana* you will be able to gauge how to combine the *asanas* to create a "meal" that is wholesome and leaves you satisfied and refreshed at the same time. While a teacher can teach you the mechanics of sequencing a routine, it is only through personal home practice that you will develop the insight necessary to fine-tune your practice to your personal needs. Nobody can tell you exactly how long to cook butter before it burns—you have to watch constantly and adjust the flame. It is only through regular practice that you can gauge how long to stay in a posture, the effect that posture has on you, and even how long to practice each day.

There are many ways to structure a hatha yoga practice, with vast differences between yoga traditions. In this chapter, I'd like to give you a way to think about practice and sequencing rather than a set of rules. The first, and perhaps the easiest, method for sequencing postures is according to their structural effects. Structural sequencing involves linking movements in an organically logical way. As you'll see, even seemingly complex postures can be broken down into a compilation of simple movements. By understanding the alphabet of movement and how motif movements form the core for families of movement, you can learn to work in a safe and thorough manner. This is a very Western way of approaching the practice, but valid nonetheless. It is the "measuring spoon" approach to cooking up your practice! The other more intuitive way of practicing, which requires greater sensitivity, is to sequence according to the energetic effects of the postures. Energetic sequencing is really the other side of the coin from structural sequencing—it involves taking the knowledge and experience you've gained from structural work and letting it *support* your intuition during your practice.

Because Westerners tend to be very focused on the appearance of things, they tend to notice only the structural effects of their practice—relaxed back muscles, looser hamstrings, or more open shoulders. But each posture also causes physiological changes in the body such as increased circulation to an organ or gland, the release of heat or toxins from a specific area, or the subtle calming of the nervous system. With practice you can learn to perceive these energetic changes. As you gain familiarity with the postures you will know how to practice to balance, stimulate, pacify, or neutralize the flow of energy in your own body.

To structure your practice from an energetic perspective requires clear perception. Energetic sequencing has less to do with increasing range of motion or practicing difficult postures, and everything to do with learning to recognize the psychophysiological effects of the postures, then deliberately orchestrating the practice to balance these effects. To work in this way it is helpful first to determine the natural proclivities of your personal constitution and those practices that stimulate, irritate, or balance you. For this I recommend that the reader consult with a reputable Ayurvedic doctor. Having a working knowledge of Ayurveda,⋆ the sister science to yoga, will help you to understand why some people feel best doing a

---

⋆Ayurveda is the ancient science and art of living in balance with nature. *Ayu* means "life," or "daily living," and *Veda* means "knowing"; thus Ayurveda means knowing how to live your life in a balanced way. I regret that this subject lies outside the scope of this book.

vigorous practice, while others thrive on gentle, slow routines. It will allow you to adapt your practice as the seasons change and as you age and your life situation changes. Respect for the needs of your individual constitution will also make it easier to avoid the pitfall of judging, comparing, or competing with others in your practice. That said, your personal constitution cannot be understood just by reading Ayurvedic theory or having someone diagnose your constitution—it still comes down to tuning in to your direct experience of how things affect you.

The knowledge of Ayurveda itself rests upon ordinary people who, through regular practice, developed extraordinary abilities to perceive the inner workings of nature—a sensitivity that you, too, can develop and hone through your own direct experiential investigation.

The following practice sequences are to help you get started. Consider them suggestions rather than strict dictates. While techniques, rules, and theories are useful guidelines, they should never tyrannize your practice. You should always honor your inner perceptions even if they fly in the face of theory. No great art, poetry, music, or culture would ever have developed if people had been slaves to rules. No master chef ever produced a sublime meal through strict adherence to measuring spoons and recipes. As you become more centered and settled into the part of your mind that is connected to its source, you will find yourself naturally choosing that which is beneficial to you. If something doesn't work for you in any of the practice sequences that follow, adapt and change it until it does. Be cautious, however, about simply avoiding postures you find challenging—they may be your most powerful and most needed medicine.

If there is one, and only one important thing that I might share with you in regard to your practice it is this: *The process of perception has no ideal and so the process of practice also has no ideal.* The Western tendency of working solely "from the head" can cause the most intelligent people to practice in ways that are neither balancing nor health promoting, and are sometimes seriously injurious. So every day, before you begin your practice, sit quietly for a few minutes and tune in to yourself. Ask yourself, "What do I need today?" Then let your practice be informed by your inner guidance. Some days this intuition may say, "I think you should sit for thirty minutes to center yourself and then do just a few quiet postures"; other days your intuition will say "Practice Sun Salutations"; and still other days it may tell you it is not good to practice at all. This deep process of listening to yourself will prevent you from being dominated by ideas, concepts, and theories, and will allow you to move from the realm of yoga as a science to yoga as an art.

THE ALPHABET OF YOGA *ASANAS*

Structural Sequencing

In the chart on page 258 (Figure 238) I have grouped postures into families of movement. At first the movements on the right of the chart might seem haphazardly grouped or seemingly unrelated, but on closer inspection you will discover they are exceedingly similar. If you turn this book on its side or upside down you'll discover that most postures are simply similar movements practiced in a different relationship to gravity. For instance, if you look at Forward Stretch (*Uttanasana*) on its side, you'll see it's remarkably similar to Stick Pose (*Dandasana*) or that Headstand (*Sirsasana*) turned right side up is Mountain Pose (*Tadasana*). Many postures belong to more than one family. East Stretch (*Purvottannasana*), for instance, is both an arm balance and a back bend and requires the essential skills of both these movement groups. Other postures are compilations of different movements around the core structure of the motif pose. Whenever you wish to learn a new posture, however seemingly complex, look at the structural components that make up the movement, and work on the essential skills of the motif movements. If you are unable to do a difficult posture on your first attempt, break down the posture into its simpler components. For instance, the skills you need to do Elbow Stand (*Pinchamayurasana*) can be acquired in Mountain Pose (which will hone your perception of your posture), Shoulder Chair Stretch (which will open your shoulders), and Downward-Facing Dog and Four-Limb Stick Pose (which build strength and flexibility in the shoulder girdle.) When you are able to do these precursor poses well, you will certainly have the skills you need to attempt Elbow Stand successfully.

The four motif movements are as follows:

Mountain Pose (*Tadasana*)

Stick Pose (*Dandasana*)

Locust Pose (*Salabhasana*)

Corpse Pose (*Savasana*)

Let's look at each motif movement and the postures that are derived from it.

from Mountain Pose *arises* . . . all standing postures and most inversions. These movements anchor the mind and ground the body, bringing you down to earth. Their practice develops strength in the legs and arms, flexibility in the hips and shoulders, and integration of the limbs with the core. They warm the body by stimulating circulation. Regular practice of these poses builds steadiness and stamina.

from Stick Pose *arises* . . . all seated movements and all seated forward bends and twists. These movements strengthen and open all the muscles on the back of the body while toning the muscles of the front of the body. They draw the circulation of blood down into the pelvis to stimulate the organs in this area. The twists squeeze and release excess

THE ALPHABET OF YOGA ASANAS

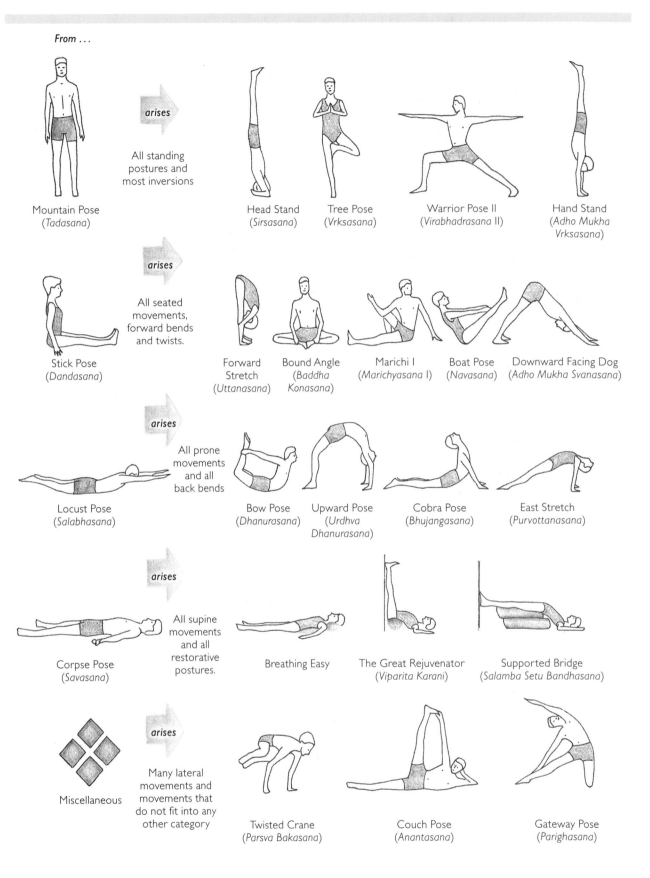

From . . .

Mountain Pose
(*Tadasana*)

arises

All standing postures and most inversions

Head Stand
(*Sirsasana*)

Tree Pose
(*Vrksasana*)

Warrior Pose II
(*Virabhadrasana* II)

Hand Stand
(*Adho Mukha Vrksasana*)

Stick Pose
(*Dandasana*)

arises

All seated movements, forward bends and twists.

Forward Stretch
(*Uttanasana*)

Bound Angle
(*Baddha Konasana*)

Marichi I
(*Marichyasana* I)

Boat Pose
(*Navasana*)

Downward Facing Dog
(*Adho Mukha Svanasana*)

Locust Pose
(*Salabhasana*)

arises

All prone movements and all back bends

Bow Pose
(*Dhanurasana*)

Upward Pose
(*Urdhva Dhanurasana*)

Cobra Pose
(*Bhujangasana*)

East Stretch
(*Purvottanasana*)

Corpse Pose
(*Savasana*)

arises

All supine movements and all restorative postures.

Breathing Easy

The Great Rejuvenator
(*Viparita Karani*)

Supported Bridge
(*Salamba Setu Bandhasana*)

Miscellaneous

arises

Many lateral movements and movements that do not fit into any other category

Twisted Crane
(*Parsva Bakasana*)

Couch Pose
(*Anantasana*)

Gateway Pose
(*Parighasana*)

FIGURE 238

heat and toxins from the internal organs and open the spine at its deepest level. Regular practice of these poses builds concentration, patience, and equipose.

from Locust Pose *arises* . . .   all prone movements (lying on the belly) and all back bends. These movements open the front of the body and strengthen the back muscles. Because they move the spine forward and open the area of the solar plexus, they tend to release heat and toxins from organs in the center of the body such as the liver and, when done with pressure on the belly, tonify the large intestine. Regular practice of these poses builds courage, tenacity, and receptivity.

from Corpse Pose *arises* . . .   all supine movements (lying on the back) and all restorative movements. These movements neutralize and balance the body and give the mind a chance to integrate the experiences of the other postures. They are calming for the nervous system and deeply rejuvenating. Regular practice of these postures develops stores of energy, increases immunity, and cultivates compassion for oneself and others.

There is a fifth category:

from Miscellaneous *arises* . . .   many lateral movements (bending to the side) and movements like arm balances that do not fit easily into any other category. These movements address often neglected areas of the body (such as the sides), or frequently neglected skills such as arm and abdominal strength. Many of these postures require keen balance, coordination, and rhythm. Their regular practice builds resourcefulness, tenacity, and imagination.

When you are beginning to practice, focus on practicing the motif postures correctly, for everything that you do or don't do in these postures will be carried over into the practice of the other movements. For instance, if you stand with your weight on your heels in Mountain Pose, it's likely you'll stand this way in every standing posture. When you've mastered the basics from the "Essential Skills" section of each of the previous *asana* chapters, you can expand your repertory of movements by first practicing the simplest derivatives of the motifs. For instance, Wide-Spread Angle (*Upavistha Konasana* I), Bound Angle (*Baddha Konasana*), and Head to Knee (*Janu Sirsasana*) are some of the most basic derivatives of Stick Pose (*Dandasana*). When these simple derivative postures are mastered, you can go on to explore more complex movements such as Revolved Head to Knee (*Parivrtta Janu Sirsasana*).

GENERAL PRACTICE

There are two main ways of working from this structural base. The first is what I call a "general" practice. In a general practice you do a few movements from each group combined with preparatory movements and stretches. This is a good way for beginners to work, because it does not strain the body by moving in one direction for too long. It also allows your body to be conditioned gradually through the synthesis of the many movements working together. For the beginner whose mind may be hard to bring to heel, the variety of many different movement challenges makes it easier to sustain focus and concentration.

THEMATIC PRACTICE

The other kind of practice is what I call a "thematic" practice. This is where you focus on a particular group of movements such as forward bends or backward bends, together with preparatory stretches and countermovements that balance or neutralize the effects of the main movement chosen. This way of practicing allows you to become very familiar with the effects of each movement and to extend your range of movement dramatically. It can, however, be more stressful on the body to emphasize one particular motion, so care should be taken not to work in an extreme or aggressive way. Thematic practices can also take the form of a psychological focus, in which you use one of the movement principles in Chapter 2 as the central focus for every posture you do.

Transitional Movements and Counterpostures

After practicing intense movements such as back bends or forward bends, it is helpful to bring the body back to a more neutral state through the use of transitional movements and counterpostures. Transitional movements are gentle movements that elongate and release the body as you are changing from one direction of movement (e.g., back bends) toward the opposite direction of movement (e.g., forward bends). They are the "neutral gear" you should pass through before moving into counterpostures. Gentle twists and movements that release the hips and elongate the back are ideal transitional movements. Counterpostures are opposing movements that take the body in exactly the opposite direction you have been working in—for instance, extending your back after prolonged flexion.

Think back to the last time you spent a few hours gardening—it doesn't take long before repeatedly bending forward begins to irritate the back and shoulders. You may find yourself naturally extending your back as you stand, or twisting to try to relieve the discomfort. While I believe counterpostures are useful, I think it is better to work in such a way that the postures do not cause compression and irritation in the first place, and if necessary to use transitional movements *before* there is irritation. Always do gentle transitional movements before counterpostures, and intersperse these movements in your practice rather than performing them only at the end of a practice. For example, when you plan to do a series of forward bends, practice a twist after every few bends rather than waiting for your back to feel tired from prolonged flexion. When you practice a series of back bends, do a few elongating movements and gentle twists after every few bends. When you do practice a counterposture, make sure you enter slowly and that you have done enough transitional movements to prepare your body.

The following are general guidelines for working with transitional movements and counterposes.

POSTURE	EXAMPLES OF TRANSITIONAL MOVEMENTS	EXAMPLES OF COUNTERPOSTURES
Forward Bends	Crossed-Legs Twist (*Parivrtta Siddhasana*) (page 161)	East Stretch (*Purvottanasana*) (page 214)
	Marichi Pose I and III (*Marichyasana* I and III) (page 166) *After forward bends you can practice more intense twists that involve extending one leg. This is because the hamstrings are already open and will not restrict the pelvis. You can work at 100% of your capacity and stay for longer duration.*	Bridge Pose (*Setu Bandhasana*) (page 194)
Back Bends	Sage Pose I and II (*Bharadvajasana* I and III) (page 164)	West Stretch (*Paschimottanasana*) (page 155)
	Reclining Big-Toe series (*Supta Padangusthasana*) (page 138) *After back bending, practice more mild twists in which both legs are bent. Back bends naturally tighten the hamstrings, and this will make the extended leg twists more challenging on your back. Go only 75% of your capacity, and stay for brief duration.*	Forward Stretch (*Uttanasana*) (page 113)
Arm Balances	Back Bend over a Bolster (page 182)	Upward-Facing Bow (*Urdhva Dhanurasana*) (page 200)
	Revolved Belly Pose (*Jathara Parivartanasana*) (page 162)	East Stretch (*Purvottanasana*) (page 214)

The following are general guidelines when working with a theme. Also, several sample general and thematic practices are offered at the end of this chapter to help you get started.

STRUCTURAL THEME	FOCUS ON PREPARATORY MOVEMENTS THAT . . .	EXAMPLES OF PREPARATORY MOVEMENTS
Forward Bends and Twists	Release your hips.	Big-Toe Reclining sequence (*Supta Padangusthasana*) (page 138)
	Open the back of your legs.	Flank Pose (*Parsvottanasana*) (page 106)
	Lengthen your spine.	Half-Dog Pose (*Ardha Svanasana*) (page 97)
Back Bends	Build heat in the body.	Sun Salutations (*Suryanamaskar*) (page 125)
	Open the fronts of your groin, belly, and chest.	Lunges and Warrior Pose I (*Virabhadrasana* I) (page 104)
	Extend your shoulders.	Elbow Stand (*Pinchamayurasana*) (page 218)
	Elongate the entire back.	Downward-Facing Dog (*Adho Mukha Svanasana*) (page 116)
	Extend your upper back.	Back Bend over bolster or ball (pages 182–87)
Arm Balances	Open your shoulders.	Shoulder Clock at wall (page 180)
	Strengthen your arms.	Four-Limb Stick Pose (*Chaturanga Dandasana*) (page 122)
	Release your hips.	Lotus Openers and Lotus Pose (*Padmasana*) (pages 150–54)
	Twist your spine.	Revolved Triangle Pose (*Parivrtta Trikonasana*) (page 108)
Inversions	Open your shoulders.	Shoulder Chair Stretch (page 181)
	Release the front of your groin.	Reclining Hero's Pose (*Supta Virasana*) (page 188)
	Lengthen your spine with particular attention to your neck.	Downward-Facing Dog with your head supported on a bolster (*Salamba Adho Mukha Svanasana*) (page 116)
Restoratives	Gently open the whole body, focusing on areas that might interfere later with your relaxation.	Slow Spinal Rolls (page 94)
	Slow the metabolic rate.	Corpse Pose (*Savasana*) (page 235)

A Core Structure for Any Practice

1. **Center the Mind and Connect to Your Breath:** Take the time *at the beginning* of your practice to feel which side of the bed you got out of that morning. Sit for at least five minutes, bringing your attention to your breath, the sensations in your body, the thoughts in your mind, and the state of your spirit. Consider what would bring balance in your practice today.

2. **Warm and Loosen:** Do a few loosening movements such as the Spinal Rolls and movements that warm the whole body, like Sun Salutations. At this stage of your practice don't work with intense specific stretches. Do movements that give a good overall effect, like Half Dog. Once the joints are lubricated, the muscles warmed, and the blood and lymph are flowing, you can proceed to the next stage.

3. **Core Practice:** Work from simple to complex, from easy to difficult, and from concrete to more subtle. Build to a climax of heat and effort, with your most challenging postures done when the body is warmest and your mind is still fresh and focused. If you are going to work on a particular type of movement like back bending, you'll want to do movements that prepare the body for that action (see chart, opposite). Also remember to practice transitional movements in between a series of back bends or forward bends to prevent strain.

4. **Cool Down and Integrate:** This is the time to practice transitional poses and counterposes such as twists after forward bends and to gradually bring your practice to a close. Always finish with Corpse Pose (*Savasana*) and/or sitting meditation to allow yourself to integrate the experience of the practice and so that you leave your practice feeling light and refreshed.

BEGINNING SEQUENCES

Each sequence takes approximately 1 hour. Alternate the sequences over the course of the week. If sitting at the beginning of your practice is too uncomfortable, try practicing that segment at the end of your session.

Practice Session A: Rise and Shine

Physical Focus: Standing Postures and Sun Salutations.
Structural Effect: Increases general strength, flexibility, and stamina.
Energetic Effect: Stimulates.

- Sitting Meditation (5 minutes) (*or alternately practice sitting before Corpse Pose, Savasana*) (page 79)
- Spinal Rolls (×3 sets, center and to both sides) (page 94)
- Sun Salutation (*Suryanamaskar*) (×3–5 rounds. Practice the variation that best suits your ability.) (page 125)
- Triangle Pose (*Trikonasana*) (×2 each side, 30 sec.–1 minute) (page 98)
- Sun Salutation (×1 round) (page 125)
- Side-Angle Pose (*Parsvakonasana*) (×2 each side, 30 sec.–1 minute) (page 100)

- Sun Salutation (×1 round)   (page 125)
- Warrior II (*Virabhadrasana* II) (×1 each side, 30 sec.–1 minute)   (page 103)
- Sun Salutation (Bring hands onto your knee during the lunge   (page 125)
  position, and slowly extend the arms over your head, 30 sec.)
- Expanded-Leg Pose (*Prasaritta Padottanasana*) (1 minute)   (page 111)
- Shoulder Stand (*Salamba Sarvangasana*) (3–5 minutes)   (page 223)
- Reclining Big-Toe Pose (*Supta Padangusthasana*)   (page 138)
  (Variation A for only 1 minute)
- Revolved Belly Pose (*Jathara Parivartanasana*) (1 minute each side) (page 162)
- Corpse Pose (*Savasana*) (5–10 minutes or more if time permits)   (page 235)

Practice Session B: Opening Up

Physical Focus: Standing Postures, Shoulder Openers, and Back Bends.
Structural Effect: Increases flexibility throughout the shoulders, back, and abdomen. Strengthens and lengthens the spine.
Energetic Effect: Releases and exhilarates.

- Sitting Meditation (5 minutes)   (page 79)
- Shoulder Clock at wall   (page 180)
- Half-Dog Pose at wall (*Ardha Svanasana*) (1 minute)   (page 97)
- Shoulder Chair Stretch (1 minute)   (page 181)
- Cow-Face Pose (*Gomukasana*)   (page 142)
  (Sitting on chair or floor—1 minute each side)
- Sun Salutation (*Suryanamaskar*) (×3–5 rounds. Emphasize your stay   (page 125)
  in the lunge and in Upward-Facing Dog.)
- Triangle Pose (*Trikonasana*) (×1 each side, 30 sec.–1 minute)   (page 98)
- Side-Angle Pose (*Parsvakonasana*) (×1 each side, 30 sec.–1 minute)   (page 100)
- Warrior I (*Virabhadrasana* I) (×1 each side, 30 sec.)   (page 104)
- Back Bend over bolster, chair, or ball   (pages 182–86)
- Locust Pose Variation A (*Salabhasana*) (×3 for 10 sec. each lift)   (page 190)
- Downward-Facing Dog (*Adho Mukha Svanasana*) (×1 for 1 minute)   (page 116)
- Locust Pose Variation B (×3 for 10 sec. each lift)   (page 191)
- Child's Pose (*Balasana*) (×1 for 1 minute)   (page 193)
- Locust Pose Variation C (×3 for 10 sec. each lift)   (page 191)
- Child's Pose (*Balasana*) (×1 for 1 minute)   (page 193)
- Bridge Pose (*Setu Bandhasana*) (×3 for 15–30 sec.)   (page 194)
- Bow Pose (*Dhanurasana*) (×1 for 15–30 sec.)   (page 195)
- Downward-Facing Dog (*Adho Mukha Svanasana*) (×1 for 1 minute)   (page 116)
- Reclining Big-Toe Pose (*Supta Padangusthasana*)   (page 138)
  (All variations for 1 minute)
- Revolved Belly Pose (*Jathara Parivartanasana*) (1 minute each side) (page 162)

• Corpse Pose with lower legs supported on chair (*Savasana*)   (page 239)
  (5 minutes or more)

Practice Session C: Turning Inward

Physical Focus: Standing Postures, Forward Bends and Twists.
Structural Effect: Releases tightness along the backs of the legs and through the spine. Strengthens the front of the body.
Energetic Effect: Cools and calms.

• Sitting Meditation (5 minutes)   (page 79)
• Spinal Rolls (×3 sets)   (page 94)
• Half-Dog Pose (*Ardha Svanasana*) (1 minute)   (page 97)
• Triangle Pose (*Trikonasana*) (×1 each side, 30 sec.–1 minute)   (page 98)
• Side-Angle Pose (*Parsvakonasana*) (×1 each side, 30 sec.–1 minute) (page 100)
• Expanded-Leg Pose (*Prasaritta Padottanasana*) (1 minute)   (page 111)
• Downward-Facing Dog (*Adho Mukha Svanasana*)   (page 116)
  (×3, 30 sec.–1 minute)
• Flank Pose with chair or block (*Parsvottanasana*)   (page 106)
  (×1 each side, 30 sec.–1 minute)
• Standing Twist with chair (×1, 1 minute each side)   (page 115)
• Forward Stretch (*Uttanasana*) (×1, 1 minute)   (page 113)
• Head-to-Knee Pose (*Janu Sirsasana*) (×1 each side, 1 minute)   (page 143)
• Wide-Spread-Angle Pose (*Upavistha Konasana*) (1 minute)   (page 146)
• Sage Pose (*Bharadvajasana* I) (×1 each side, 1 minute)   (page 164)
• Marichi Pose I (*Marichyasana* I) (×1 each side, 1 minute)   (page 166)
• Bound-Angle Pose (*Baddha Konasana*)   (page 148)
  (1 minute sitting, 1 minute forward bending)
• West Stretch (*Paschimottanasana*) (1 minute)   (page 155)
• Revolved Belly Pose (*Jathara Parivartanasana*)   (page 162)
  (×1 each side, 1 minute)
• The Great Rejuvenator (*Viparita Karani*)   (page 245)
  (5–10 minutes)
• Corpse Pose (*Savasana*) (3–5 minutes)   (page 235)

Practice Session D: Returning

Physical Focus: Supported Restorative and Breathing Practices.
Structural Effect: Releases tension throughout the entire body.
Energetic Effect: Centers, soothes, and rejuvenates.

- Spinal Rolls (×3 practiced very slowly)   (page 94)
- Supported Forward Bend (3–5 minutes)   (page 240)
  Choose *two* from the following and practice with head supported on a chair:
  - ~ Tailor's Pose   (page 141)
  - ~ Head-to-Knee Pose (*Janu Sirsasana*)   (page 143)
  - ~ Wide-Spread-Angle Pose I and II (*Upavistha Konasana* I and II)   (page 146)
- Supported Bound-Angle Pose (*Salamba Supta Baddha Konasana*)   (page 243)
  (5 minutes)
- The Great Rejuvenator (*Viparita Karani*) (5–10 minutes)   (page 245)
- Downward-Facing Corpse Pose (*Adho Mukha Savasana*)   (page 239)
  (5–10 minutes)
  Or Corpse Pose variation of your choice (*Savasana*)   (page 239)
- Breathing Practices
  Choose *one* from the following:
  - ~ Straw Breathing (3–5 minutes)   (page 247)
  - ~ The Pacifying Breath (*Viloma* II) (3–5 minutes)   (page 249)
  - ~ The Purifying Breath (*Nadi Shodhanam*) (3–5 minutes)   (page 248)
- Simple Sitting Meditation (5–15 minutes)   (page 79)

INTERMEDIATE/ADVANCED SEQUENCES

*These practices take approximately 1½ to 2 hours depending on the length of your beginning medita-
tion. Alternate the sequences over the course of a week. Practice the modified variations of poses you
find difficult, rather than skipping them altogether. Postures designated with a ☆ are optional.*

Practice Session A: Rise and Shine

Physical Focus: Standing Postures and Sun Salutations.
Structural Effect: Increases general strength, flexibility, and stamina.
Energetic Effect: Stimulates.

- Sitting Meditation (5–30 minutes)   (page 79)
- Spinal Rolls (×3 sets, center and to both sides)   (page 94)
- Sun Salutation/Standing Posture (*Vinyasana*)   (page 128)
  Insert these standing postures inside the cycle:
  - ~ Triangle Pose (*Trikonasana*) (×1 each side, 1 minute)   (page 98)
  - ~ Side-Angle Pose (*Parsvakonasana*) (×1 each side, 1 minute)   (page 100)
  - ~ Warrior II (*Virabhadrasana* II) (×1 each side, 1 minute)   (page 103)
  - ~ Warrior I (*Virabhadrasana* I) (×1 each side, 1 minute)   (page 104)
  - ~ Half-Moon Pose (*Ardha Chandrasana*) (×1 each side, 1 minute)   (page 110)
- Expanded-Leg Pose (*Prasaritta Padottanasana*) (2 minutes)   (page 111)

☆ Headstand (*Salamba Sirsasana*) (3–7 minutes) (page 220)

• Shoulder Stand (*Salamba Sarvangasana*) (3–7 minutes) (page 223)

• Reclining Big-Toe Pose (*Supta Padangusthasana*) (page 138)
  (All variations 1 minute)

• Revolved Belly Pose (*Jathara Parivartanasana*) (1 minute each side) (page 162)

• Corpse Pose (*Savasana*) (5–10 minutes or more if time permits) (page 235)

Practice Session B: Opening Up

Physical Focus: Arm Balances, Shoulder Openers, and Back Bends.

Structural Effect: Increases flexibility throughout the shoulders, back, and abdomen. Strengthens and lengthens the spine.

Energetic Effect: Releases and lightens.

• Sitting Meditation sitting in Hero's Pose (5 minutes) (page 79)

• Reclining Hero/Heroine's Pose (*Supta Virasana*) (page 188)

• Horseman's Pose (*Uktasana*) (At the beginning of each Sun Salutation) (page 96)

• Sun Salutation (*Suryanamaskar*) (×5–10 rounds. (page 125)
  Emphasize your stay in the lunge and in Upward-Facing Dog)

☆ Handstand (*Adho Mukha Vrksasana*) (×1–3 for 15–30 sec.) (page 216)

☆ Elbow Stand (*Pinchamayurasana*) (×1–3 for 15–30 sec.) (page 218)

• Back Bend over bolster, chair, or ball (pages 182–86)

• Cobra Pose (*Bhujangasana*) (×3 for 15–30 sec.) (page 198)

• Bow Pose (*Dhanurasana*) (×3 for 15–30 sec.) (page 195)

• Child's Pose (*Balasana*) (1 minute) (page 193)

• Camel Pose (*Ustrasana*) (×3 for 15–30 sec.) (page 196)

• Upward-Facing Bow (*Urdhva Dhanurasana*) (×3 for 15–30 sec.) (page 200)

• Downward-Facing Dog (*Adho Mukha Svanasana*) (×1 for 1 minute) (page 116)

• Sage Pose I and II (*Bharadvajasana* I and II) (×1 each side for 1 minute) (page 164)

• West Stretch (*Paschimottanasana*) (1–3 minutes) (page 155)

• Revolved Belly Pose (*Jathara Parivartanasana*) (1 minute each side) (page 162)

• Corpse Pose (*Savasana*) (5–10 minutes) (page 235)

Practice Session C: Turning Inward

Physical Focus: Standing Postures, Forward Bends, and Twists.

Structural Effect: Releases tightness along the backs of the legs and through the spine. Strengthens the front of the body.

Energetic Effect: Cools and calms.

• Sitting Meditation (5–30 minutes) (page 79)

• Reclining Big-Toe Pose (*Supta Padangusthasana*) (page 138)
  (1 minute each position)

- Through-the-Hole Stretch (1–3 minutes each side) (page 150)
- Head-to-Knee Pose (*Janu Sirsasana*) (×2 each side, 3 minutes) (page 143)
- Half Lotus Forward Bend (*Ardha Baddha Padma Paschimottasana*) (page 152)
  (×1 each side, 3 minutes)
- Sage Pose II (*Bharadvajasana* II) (×1 each side, 1 minute) (page 164)
- Wide-Spread-Angle Pose I and II (*Upavistha Konasana* I and II) (page 146)
  (1 minute)
- Lotus Opener Series (Choose two: 1 minute each position) (page 150)
- ☆ Lotus Pose (*Padmasana*) (1–5 minutes) (page 154)
- Marichi Pose III (*Marichyasana* III) (×1 each side, 1 minute) (page 168)
- Lord of the Fishes (*Ardha Matsyendrasana*) (page 169)
  (×1 each side, 1 minute)
- West Stretch (*Paschimottanasana*) (3 minutes) (page 155)
- Shoulder Stand (*Salamba Sarvangasana*) (5–7 minutes) (page 223)
- Revolved Belly Pose (*Jathara Parivartanasana*) (page 162)
  (×1 each side, 1 minute)
- Corpse Pose (*Savasana*) (5–10 minutes) (page 235)

Practice Session D: Inner Power

Physical Focus: Arm Balances and Inversions.
Structural Effect: Strengthens and releases the arms and shoulders. Tonifies the abdominal muscles and all the muscles of the trunk.
Energetic Effect: Tonifies and strengthens organ and glandular function. Balances the nervous system.

- Sitting Meditation (Kneeling in Hero's Pose) (5 minutes) (page 188)
- Cow-Face Pose (*Gomukasana*) (×2 each side for 1 minute) (page 142)
- Reclining Hero/Heroine's Pose (*Supta Virasana*) (3–5 minutes) (page 188)
- Downward-Facing Dog (*Adho Mukha Svanasana*) (1–3 minutes) (page 116)
- One-Arm Stand (*Vasisthasana*) (30 sec.–1 minute each side) (page 214)
- East Stretch (*Purvottanasana*) (1 minute) (page 214)
- Shoulder Chair Stretch (1–3 minutes) (page 181)
- Elbow Stand (*Pinchamayurasana*) (×3 for 30 sec.–1 minute) (page 218)
- Forward Stretch (*Uttanasana*) (1–3 minutes) (page 113)
- Headstand (*Salamba Sirsasana*) (3–7 minutes) (page 220)
- Plow Pose (*Halasana*) (3–5 minutes) (page 226)
- Shoulder Stand (*Salamba Sarvangasana*) (3–7 minutes) (page 223)
- Knee-to-Ear Pose (*Karnapidasana*) (3–5 minutes) (page 228)
- Revolved Belly Pose (*Jathara Parivartanasana*) (page 162)
  (1–3 minutes each side)
- Corpse Pose (*Savasana*) (5–10 minutes) (page 235)

Practice Session E: Returning

Physical Focus: Supported Restorative and Breathing Practices.
Structural Effect: Releases tension throughout the entire body.
Energetic Effect: Centers, soothes, and rejuvenates.

- Simple Sitting Meditation (15–30 minutes) (Sitting may (page 79)
  alternatively be practiced at the end of the practice session)
- Big-Toe Pose: all variations (*Supta Padangusthasana*) (1 minute each) (page 138)
- Supported Forward Bend (3–5 minutes) (page 240)
  Choose *two* from the following and practice with head supported on a chair:
  - ∼ Head-to-Knee Pose (*Janu Sirsasana*) (page 143)
  - ∼ Half Lotus Forward Bend (*Ardha Baddha* (page 152)
    Padma Paschimottanasana)
  - ∼ Wide-Spread-Angle Pose I and II (*Upavistha Konasana* I and II) (page 146)
- Supported Bound-Angle Pose (*Salamba Supta Baddha Konasana*) (page 243)
  (5 minutes)
- The Great Rejuvenator (*Viparita Karani*) (5–10 minutes) (page 245)
- Breathing Practices or sitting if you did not do so (pages 79)
  at the beginning of the practice.
  Choose *one* from the following:
  - ∼ Straw Breathing (5–7 minutes) (page 247)
  - ∼ The Pacifying Breath (*Viloma* II) (5–7 minutes) (page 249)
  - ∼ The Purifying Breath (*Nadi Shodhanam*) (5–7 minutes) (page 248)
- Corpse Pose (*Savasana*) (5–10 minutes) (page 235)

Notes

CHAPTER ONE

1. *Effortless Being, The Yoga Sutras of Patanjali* trans. Alistair Shearer (London: Unwin Paperbacks, 1982; reprint, 1989), 32.
2. I credit this very original way of looking at the sutras to a talk given by Richard Miller, Ph.D, November 1998 at Kripalu Center's "Yoga on the Leading Edge" retreat.
3. Pema Chödrön, *When Things Fall Apart* (Boston: Shambhala Publications, 1996).

CHAPTER TWO

1. Swami Satyananda Saraswati and Swami Muktibodhananda Saraswati, *Swara Yoga: Tantric Science of Brain Breathing,* Published by Sri G. K. Kejriwal, Honorary Secretary, Bihar School of Yoga. Printed and Distributed by: Satyananda Ashram, Australia, Mangrove Mountain, R.M.B. 4820, Gosford, N.S.W. 2250, Australia, 1983,. page 4.
2. For further reading on human developmental movement patterns, see "Sensing, Feeling and Action" Bonnie Bainbridge Cohen, Contact Editions, MA, 1993.
3. Rene Cailliet, M.D., *Low Back Pain Syndrome,* 3rd ed. (Philadelphia: Davis, 1981), 7.
4. The work of Bonnie Bainbridge Cohen, director of the School for Body-Mind Centering, has emerged as one of the most relevant somatic practices for modern-day yogis. Through her work and the experiential research of hundreds of students over the course of more than twenty-five years, we now have a basic model for accessing a deeper somatic understanding of ourselves. The basic premise of the work is that by watching the movement of the body, we can see the movement of the mind. Integral to this understanding is the uncompromising belief that consciousness pervades *all* the body. The study of BMC includes, but is not limited to, a cognitive and experiential learning of the body systems—skeleton, ligaments, muscles, fascia, fat, skin, organs, endocrine glands, nerves, fluids, breathing, the senses and dynamics of perception, human developmental movement patterns, and the art of touch and repatterning.
5. Discussions with Lynne Uretsky, certified Body-Mind Centering instructor, 1996. Her original statement was as follows: "The cellular level of awareness is the field from which all other intentions form."
6. For a fascinating discussion of the chemical composition of bone, see Henry Gray, *Gray's Anatomy,* (New York: Bounty Books, 1101).
7. Gerard Tortora and Nicholas Anagnostakos, *Principles of Anatomy and Physiology* (New York: Harper & Row, 1984), 130.

8. Arthur Guyton and John Hall, *Textbook of Medical Physiology,* (Philadelphia: W. B Saunders, 1996), 991.

9. Dio Urmilla Neff, "The Great Chakra Controversy," *Yoga Journal* (November/December 1985): 42–45.

10. The coccygeal body is not shown in most anatomy texts. An illustration can be seen in *Anatomy: A Regional Atlas of the Human Body,* 3rd ed. (Munich: Urban and Schwarzenberg, 1987), Plate 377.

11. M. G. Nicholls, "Editorial and Historical Review," in Mini-symposium: "The Natriuretic Peptide Hormones," *Journal of Internal Medicine* 235 (1994): 507; and Harriet MacMillan and Meir Steiner, "Commentary: Atrial Natriuretic Factor: Does It Have a Role in Psychiatry?" *Biological Psychiatry* 35 (1994): 272–77.

CHAPTER FIVE

1. The pivotal role of the hyoid was first introduced to me through the work of Jim Spira at the now defunct Institute for Educational Therapy in Berkeley, California. Its relationship to the digestive and respiratory function has been further clarified through discussions with staff from the School for Body-Mind Centering.

CHAPTER SIX

1. The classification of Headstand as an *asana* appears to be relatively recent, contends yoga scholar Georg Feuerstein, who provided me with background material for my original research of Headstand in 1993.

2. The *sushumna* is considered one of three chief pathways for the movement of life force through the body. The yogin's challenge is to direct the flow of energy through this bioenergetic conduit, stabilizing and potentiating the nervous system at once. To the left of this axial pathway lies the *ida-nadi* and to the right the *pingala-nadi*. The *ida-nadi* is symbolized by the lunar, or cooling, element and is related to the parasympathetic branch of the nervous system. The *pingala-nadi* is symbolized by the sun, or warming, element and is related to the sympathetic branch of the nervous system. When the "sun" and "moon" (the word *hatha* is literally translated as sun/moon) elements are perfectly balanced the movement of energy is centralized through the *sushumna*. This centralization of the movement of energy through this powerful channel, commonly referred to as *kundalini* energy, is believed to give the practitioner access to tremendous energetic powers which, if used correctly, lead to a transcendental consciousness.

3. Judith Lasater, *Relax and Renew* (Berkeley, Calif.: Rodmell Press, 1995), 158.

CHAPTER SEVEN

1. N. Vijayan, M.D., "Head Band for Migraine Headache Relief," *Headache* 33, no. 1 (January 1993): 40–41.

2. This exercise is adapted from Carola Speads, *Ways to Better Breathing* (Rochester, Vt.: Healing Arts Press, 1992).

3. The following present evidence supporting nostril dominance and its effect on the nervous system: Ernest Lawrence Rossi, with David Nimmons, *The Twenty-Minute Break: Using the New Science of Ultradian Rhythms* (Los Angeles: Jeremy Tarcher, 1991); and David Shannahoff-Khalsa, "Lateralized Rhythms of the Central and Autonomic Nervous System," *International Journal of Psychophysiology,* 11, no. 3 (1991): 222–51.

Yoga with Donna Farhi

∼

For Donna Farhi's international teaching itinerary and for information on workshops, retreats, and yoga teacher training programs, visit her Web site:

www.donnafarhi.co.nz